UNINSURED IN CHICAGO

Uninsured in Chicago

How the Social Safety Net Leaves Latinos Behind

Robert Vargas

NEW YORK UNIVERSITY PRESS

New York

NEW YORK UNIVERSITY PRESS
New York
www.nyupress.org

References to Internet websites (URLs) were accurate at the time of writing. Neither the author nor New York University Press is responsible for URLs that may have expired or changed since the manuscript was prepared.

Library of Congress Cataloging-in-Publication Data
Names: Vargas, Robert, 1985– author.
Title: Uninsured in Chicago : how the social safety net leaves Latinos behind / Robert Vargas.
Description: New York : New York University Press, [2022] | Series: Latina/o sociology | Includes bibliographical references and index.
Identifiers: LCCN 2021039791 | ISBN 9781479807130 (hardback ; alk. paper) | ISBN 9781479807147 (paperback ; alk. paper) | ISBN 9781479807161 (ebook) | ISBN 9781479807260 (ebook other)
Subjects: LCSH: United States. Patient Protection and Affordable Care Act. | Hispanic Americans—Medical care—Illinois—Chicago—Case studies. | Hispanic Americans—Health and hygiene—Illinois—Chicago—Case studies. | Health insurance—Illinois—Chicago—Case studies. | Medical care—Illinois—Chicago—Case studies.
Classification: LCC RA412.475 .V37 2022 | DDC 368.38/200977311—dc23
LC record available at https://lccn.loc.gov/2021039791

New York University Press books are printed on acid-free paper, and their binding materials are chosen for strength and durability. We strive to use environmentally responsible suppliers and materials to the greatest extent possible in publishing our books.

Manufactured in the United States of America

10 9 8 7 6 5 4 3 2 1

Also available as an ebook

CONTENTS

Introduction

"I'm sorry if you can't hear me well," said soft-spoken Nick Rodriguez. A 28-year-old uninsured Mexican American, Nick suffered from severe asthma, and his voice was faint in our first interview. It was January 2013, and we sat in an otherwise empty McDonald's in Chicago's Little Village neighborhood. The Affordable Care Act (ACA) had gone into effect just a few weeks earlier.

"I've been in the emergency room a couple times," Nick said. "Sometimes I just wake up purple, like I can't breathe, can't even talk. So, my girl would have to call the ambulance for me and that's scary."

"Have you ever tried to get health insurance?" I asked.

"Yeah," Nick responded, clarifying, "It's where they give you benefits and help to get medicine—stuff like that?"

"Yeah. Have you applied for it?" I asked again.

"Yeah, I've applied for health insurance before, but I've gotten denied. In the past they've said that asthma is not . . . how do you call it . . . covered."

"So, what do you do when you have an asthma attack?"

"I end up going to the University Hospital emergency room."

"Have they been charging you?"

"Yeah, I got all my bills. It's ridiculous. A lot of money."

"Roughly how much?"

"Oh my god, probably more than $60,000. Pretty sure more than that."

"Did you ever think about going to Stroger hospital [the county hospital], whenever you've had your asthma attacks? It might be cheaper there."

"Yes, I did, but to be honest, I don't go there because there is a wait there. I wait a lot there. And once I go to my hospital, once I get there, I get a room right away. I don't even have to wait five, ten minutes. If I go over here, I have to wait at least four, five hours."

"What do you know about the Affordable Care Act?"

"Is that the Obama?"

"It is. It's also called Obamacare. Yeah. Do you think you'll try to get it?"

"Right now, I don't trust them. I just want to see what happens. I want to hear people saying, 'Oh, they're helping me with my bills, with my medicine.' I want to see somebody who got it."

* * *

In 2013, roughly half of US Latino young adults between the ages of 18 and 34 were uninsured, a problem the ACA was supposed to help fix. The ACA represented an enormous shift in health care governance, and its provisions opened unprecedented opportunities for Latinos to acquire health insurance. Among its best-known effects, the ACA allowed young adults to stay on their parents' health insurance until age 26, prevented insurers from denying coverage to people with preexisting conditions, expanded Medicaid eligibility to single able-bodied adults between 18 and 64 who earned under 138% of the federal poverty level, and created state marketplaces in which uninsured individuals (ineligible for Medicaid) could purchase private insurance with the help of a government subsidy. Modeled after Republican governor Mitt Romney's health care reform in Massachusetts, the ACA treated health care as a commodity and not a human right. Thus, like car insurance, the ACA mandated citizens to purchase private health insurance or enroll in Medicaid.

So why didn't millions of uninsured Latinos like Nick actually enroll? This troubling trend has puzzled scholars, policymakers, and health care providers. Of the ACA's many provisions, Medicaid expansion was key for Latinos, the highest percent uninsured group in the nation.[1] Millions of previously ineligible Latinos could apply for this government health insurance program for low-income people.[2] Six years after implementation, they hadn't: Latinos turned out to be the racial group least likely to enroll.[3] Enormous sums were poured into advertising campaigns, and the percentage of uninsured Latinos decreased from 15.7% in 2013 to 9.1% in 2019, yet a total of 10.1 million now-eligible US Latinos remained uninsured (half of them millennials aged 18 to 35 years old, 59% male and 41% female).[4]

This is, to put it mildly, a major problem. Health insurance brings enormous benefits that many Latinos need. In addition to facilitating access to medical services, health insurance protects individuals and families from financial ruin.[5] In 2013 alone, 2 million personal bankruptcy filings were attributed to unpaid medical bills, outpacing both credit card debt and unpaid mortgages.[6] For Latino families just one medical emergency away from financial disaster, health insurance coverage has the potential to foster economic well-being. Lacking such coverage is a major driver of Latinos' economic precarity.

The brutal four-year presidency of Donald J. Trump significantly worsened the problem. President Trump's racist caricatures of Latinos expanded and hardened immigration enforcement, and the detention of migrant adults and children at the US–Mexico border has had a chilling effect on Latino Medicaid enrollment. The concurrent resurgence of anti-Latino racism underscored the imperative to improve Latino participation in health insurance programs and government programs more generally,[7] yet scholars and industry experts agree that fewer Latinos, particularly those who lived in counties with stricter immigration enforcement policies, sought enrollment under the Trump administration.[8] Trump's four invective-filled years in office are over; still, the consequences of his anti-immigrant and anti-Latino postures and policies will prove difficult for any future administration to remedy.

Even more troubling, Latinos' low participation rates in government programs are not limited to Medicaid or health insurance programs. Despite higher levels of poverty, Latinos also have the lowest rates of participation in public assistance programs such as Temporary Assistance for Needy Families and Supplemental Nutrition Assistance Program.[9] This matters tremendously for policy efforts aimed at expanding the nation's social safety net. For example, a group led by Latina congresswoman Alexandria Ocasio-Cortez has introduced the "Green New Deal," a massive federal reinvestment act aimed at addressing climate change that would create higher-paying jobs and improve access to food, health care, and housing. Without a deeper understanding of Latinos' low participation rates, those seeking to strengthen the social safety net are unlikely to bring Latinos into the fold. The logic of "If you build it, Latinos will come" does not apply to social policy.

The scant social science on Latinos' low program participation rates has pointed to a number of possible explanations; however, none is sufficient. Some surveys and interview studies suggest that Latinos are often unaware of their eligibility or believe "they don't need" such supports.[10] Other studies point to immigration status, with fearful Latino immigrant families describing a desire to avoid potentially disclosing their undocumented status to any government agency—and reaping disastrous consequences.

* * *

This book tells the stories of uninsured Latinos' experience with the ACA in Chicago. I aim to answer what seems, on the surface, a straightforward question: *Why did some uninsured Latino millennials enroll in Medicaid while others did not?*

I engaged in a longitudinal ethnographic study of the uninsured, shadowing 25 Latinos, nine African Americans, and six whites during the first three years of ACA implementation (2013–16). I observed my participants as they lived their daily lives, messaged with them on social media, and accompanied them as they sought information about the ACA or interacted with the health care system. Chicago proved an ideal site for this study: 44% of the Chicagoland area's total Medicaid-eligible population—some 681,000 individuals—remained uninsured from 2014 to 2016.[11] This was one of the most Democratic and pro-Obama areas of the country, yet 40% of African Americans and 30% of Latinos who became eligible for Medicaid here did not enroll.[12]

I identified and recruited participants from four Chicago neighborhoods: Humboldt Park, Little Village, Logan Square, and North Lawndale. I chose these neighborhoods because Humboldt Park (57%) and Little Village (83%) were majority Latino and had among the highest rates of uninsured individuals in Chicago (21% and 29%, respectively).[13] Humboldt Park's median income was $34,315, while Little Village was $30,701. I included North Lawndale and Logan Square to incorporate African Americans and whites into my study sample. North Lawndale is a majority Black neighborhood with a median income of $26,781. Although Logan Square has more recently gentrified, at the time of this study (2013–16), its median income was $56,165, and it was home to a considerable population of uninsured lower-middle-class whites.

My data collection took place long before the COVID-19 pandemic, yet the 60623 zip code spanning North Lawndale and Little Village (shown in figure I.1) would come to have the city's highest rates of CO-VID-19 infections and deaths.[14] During my study, the 60623 zip code was 60% Latino and 32% African American, and it had the city's highest rate of uninsurance.[15] As of December 2020, 170 Latinos have died from COVID-19 in just this postal code. Sadly, national-level racial disparities in COVID-19 infections and deaths have proved durable through the first year of the pandemic. Because Latinos make up a large share of the essential (but often low-wage) workforce and have higher rates of preexisting health conditions, COVID-19 has inflicted almost unimaginable harm on the Latino population. While this group makes up just 18% of the nation's population, in December 2020, they accounted for a shocking 23.4% of its COVID-19 infections and 32.9% of its COVID-19 deaths.[16]

And these numbers are likely a severe undercount. An unknown number of Latinos went without medical care after developing COVID-like symptoms, a wariness Dr. Eva Galvez of the Migrant Clinicians Network attributes to a combined lack of health insurance and mistrust and fear of government.[17] Thus, while this book is based on data collected prior to the pandemic, the stories I share about Latinos' reluctance to

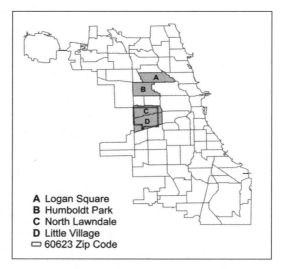

FIGURE I.I. Map of Chicago Neighborhoods Sample.
Source: Christina Cano.

enroll in Medicaid offer insight into why so many Latinos may have foregone COVID-19 tests and treatment—and why they may forego vaccination.

My longitudinal, ethnographic approach illuminated more complete and complex explanations for uninsured Latinos' reluctance to apply for Medicaid than previous studies have been able to access. Nick Rodriguez is a prime example. Had I stopped collecting data after that first interview at the Little Village McDonalds, I may have concluded that Nick's past experience with private insurance or the county hospital had soured his perceptions of Medicaid. Instead, by shadowing Nick over the course of three years, I was able to observe even more powerful reasons for his reluctance. Nick was purchasing asthma inhalers from his neighborhood's informal economy and generating the income to do so by shoplifting. After a year, Nick was caught, convicted, and imprisoned for a year, which amplified his unease when it came to applying for government benefits (chapter 1 dives deeper into Nick's experience). It took time and trust for me to detangle the social structures that inhibit uninsured Latinos' Medicaid participation, including, in Nick's case, the criminalization of informal health care economies.

Certainly, a longitudinal ethnographic approach is not without limitations. It sacrifices breadth for depth. I intentionally sought to delve deeper into the lives of fewer uninsured individuals so that I could investigate the experiences contributing to their reluctance to enroll in Medicaid. This means, however, that my findings cannot be interpreted as representative of the experience for all Latinos or all uninsured people in the United States. At the same time, this book suggests new approaches and questions for scholars and policymakers to pursue in an effort to improve Latino participation in government programs, including Medicaid.

Overall, the findings in these pages point to four understudied social structures that, I argue, could be fruitfully transformed to improve Latino Medicaid participation. Down the line, meaningful engagement with these issues might even raise the standard of living and quality of life for millions and millions of Americans, Latinos included. These social structures are (1) the criminalized informal health care economy, (2) racialized bureaucracies, (3) gendered family dynamics, and (4) college networks.

First, the criminalized informal health care economy represents an oppressive binding of the criminal justice and health care systems. In the absence of universal health insurance, informal economies emerge to fill the needs of the uninsured population (for instance, prescription medications and medical equipment). When uninsured Latinos and African Americans turn to this informal economy, it means risking punishment under a criminal justice system that does not distinguish the sale of heroin from the sale of asthma inhalers. Thus, the health care and criminal justice systems converge in low-income, underinsured Latino and African American neighborhoods, and the resulting disproportionate incarceration of both groups traps them in a cycle of poverty when their criminal record impedes future employment prospects.

Second, racialized bureaucracies deeply influence Latinos' reluctance or enthusiasm toward applying for Medicaid.[18] For many in this study, their first impression of the health care safety net came in the form of a visit to a county clinic, emergency room, or state public aid office. Their bureaucratic interactions often resulted in Latinos enduring long waits, rude and indifferent treatment, and stigmatization—all of which racialized the uninsured by teaching them that they were not deserving of government assistance with health care. Such traumatic experiences had a chilling effect on respondents' interest in applying for Medicaid or securing private insurance with ACA subsidies.[19] It's worth noting that some uninsured Latinos describe positive memories, including receiving lifesaving low-cost medical assistance for a serious health emergency, and these respondents were comfortable with and eager to apply for Medicaid when the ACA was implemented. The difference represents the potential of humane and respectful public benefit provision to help uninsured Latinos.

Third, gendered family dynamics produce unique barriers to Medicaid enrollment for Latinos and Latinas. Job growth in the United States has been concentrated in the low-wage service sector, and so huge numbers of Latino millennials continue to live at home with their parents even after finishing college. Consequently, many have remained on a parent's employer-provided family health insurance plan. As the ACA increased the maximum age that young adults can remain on their parents' health insurance plan (from 23 to 26 years old), the ACA has turned the process of seeking insurance into one marked by the uneven prioritization of sons' and daughters' needs and desires. In my sample, uninsured Latina women were significantly more constrained by their parents than were their uninsured male counterparts. Patriarchal family structures privileged their men's health care needs and financial independence over women's. As family, labor market, and health care structures have become increasingly intertwined, gender looms large, producing unique constraints on Medicaid access for Latina women and Latino men.

Finally, college networks play a key role in disseminating information about the ACA to a large number of uninsured Latino and African American young adults, who are increasingly entering community colleges and four-year universities. College campuses have become critical sites of information sharing among classmates and roommates, and health insurance information is no exception. ACA outreach efforts were targeted accordingly, and the first year of ACA implementation involved blanketing Chicago's campuses with flyers and hosting on-site workshops about the process of acquiring—or helping others acquire—the health insurance for which they were newly eligible.

By describing how these interdependent social structures facilitate and constrain Latinos' participation in Medicaid, this book aims to guide the attention of those interested in expanding Latinos' health care access toward key sites for intervention. Devising policies and outreach strategies that take the informal economy, the family, bureaucracy, and campus networks seriously may generate new approaches to boosting Latino health insurance enrollment, and it will improve our understandings of how race, class, and gender shape the lives of Latinos in the twenty-first century. It is my hope that readers will imagine new ways to empower communities to rethink, redesign, rebuild, and repurpose these social structures for the better.

While the book is focused largely on Latinos, the framework and methodology employed may be fruitful for generating deeper insights on access to health care or other benefit programs for other marginalized groups. Readers more interested in findings than theory, I suggest, should move ahead, diving right into chapter 1, and those seeking a discussion of the study's implications and my suggested solutions can skip to the concluding chapter. The remainder of this introduction goes into greater depth on the intersectional theoretical framework undergirding my ethnographic approach—and my recommendations.

Boosting Latino Enrollment

This book's approach to the study of the uninsured is grounded in an intersectional theoretical framework, which I apply to analyze the social structures inhibiting Latino access to Medicaid and public benefits more generally. This approach works differently than standard policy research approaches, which tend to focus on changing individual behavior. Social change, not exclusively policy prescription, is the aim of intersectional research.

A focus on social change is especially urgent in this moment: the Trump presidency has reminded researchers that we cannot assume that policymakers or philanthropic leaders respect science or are capable of persuasion or that well-intentioned social provision programs are politically neutral, equally accessible, or universally desired. These times require social justice–oriented social scientists to approach our research with goals that go beyond identifying individual risk factors and translating them into granular policy contributions. We must also identify and explain the connections that bind oppressive social structures so that social movements and civic organizations might transform them.[20]

An intersectional approach to Latino Medicaid enrollment involved specifying the places, situations, and interactions in which social structures converge to shape health care decision-making.[21] Applying this framework renders a more complete picture of uninsured Latinos and the multiple structures they navigate when seeking health insurance. It provides researchers an alternative epistemology from which to ethnographically study marginalized Latinos. And in contrast to approaches that focus exclusively on description or storytelling meant to evoke emotive responses in predominantly white readers—critiqued as "poverty porn" or "jungle book" ethnography—the intersectional approach engages the researcher in intelligence gathering and knowledge production to inform the actions of community members, social service agencies, and social movements.[22]

The power of this approach comes from its unparalleled capacity to identify how systems of oppression intersect.[23] Specifically, I rely on sociologist Patricia Hill-Collins's method for applying intersectional theory to ethnographic data. Hill-Collins urges researchers to focus on "the places that connect various parts,"[24] a particularly generative instruction for Latino health care researchers.[25] Over the course of my fieldwork, this analytical lens allowed me to tease out the social structures that, in combination, influence uninsured Latinos' decision-making. Attending to their convergences significantly advances insights into my respondents' social worlds and points to innovative ideas for producing social change.[26]

My intersectional approach in this book is necessary for advancing beyond the limitations of existing studies on Latino health insurance enrollment.[27] Based largely on interview, survey, or administrative data, other researchers have done an excellent job describing risk factors and barriers to enrollment, yet they have offered little insight regarding how to empower Latinos themselves to overcome or transform the ties that bind. This limitation, of course, has less to do with individual researcher motivations than the inherent limitations of the factor-based research designs taught in schools of public policy or public health and applied in past studies of Latino health insurance.[28]

Adopting the intersectional framework advances the field in several ways. First, it can help provide Latino communities with strategic intelligence for acquiring benefits from a complex and often hostile social safety net. To be clear, I don't mean "intelligence" as individual IQ but as the strategic application of knowledge. Rather than waiting for government officials to change policy, providing strategic intelligence to those who could benefit from policy can help empower uninsured Latinos in their efforts to seek care while also avoiding harmful social structures. For example, intelligence gathered from studying the operation of the health care safety net and the ways government shapes Latino communities can become *strategic* intelligence aimed at helping Latinos overcome fear of the state by sharing information for navigating the state safely.

Some might question my use of the term "intelligence" in this context. These words bring to mind warfare. And they are meant to. I'd argue that the migrant detention camps, immigration enforcement raids, and racist messages put forth by the government toward and about Latinos effectively amount to a war being waged against US Latino communities. While policy researchers often operate with the assumption that elected officials can be convinced by evidence and data, the intersectional social scientist's objectives are centered on providing Latino communities with the knowledge needed to navigate the current system, accessing state beneficence while avoiding its many potential harms.[29]

Community-based health organizations, which have designed and implemented some of the most successful interventions for improving Latino access to health care, are best positioned to make use of this knowledge.[30] Conducting research with an intersectional approach can be thought of as constructing a topographical map for organizers, activists, and advocates, noting potential landmines and safe harbors. This is the sort of intelligence that enables communities to identify, change, evade, resist, or subvert hazardous social structures.

Intersectional researchers also have greater flexibility to explore and discover influential social structures that may be obscured by relying only on previously asked questions or administrative data.[31] For example, the literature points to fear of immigration enforcement authorities as a key barrier to Latinos accessing Medicaid (especially for Mexican Americans). While fear is important, it is just one of many possible ways that Latinos' relationship with government can influence health insurance enrollment.[32] Moreover, what exactly is the "fear" that Mexican Americans are experiencing? How is it overcome? And how can civic groups best respond to those fears? The fragmented, multilayered, and multiagency form of US government suggests that fear likely operates in complex and nuanced ways that may hinder or help Latinos depending on the time, place, or presence of other social structures.

This theoretical foundation opens up the possibility for researchers to discover a wider *set* of mechanisms at play in producing the same outcomes. That is, using the example of Latinos' avoidance of government programs like Medicaid, we can start to see that fear is only one possible reason for that avoidance. Rational abstention is certainly as likely a motivation, and qualitative research on poor people's politics has demonstrated that the decision to forego Medicaid can stem from disdain for a government perceived to be paternalistic, punitive, or invasive of privacy.[33] Amid many possible ways that Latinos can relate to the state and to individual state agencies, fear of immigration enforcement has been foregrounded, while possibilities including rational abstention or a wider exploration of how uninsured Latinos perceive the state and its health care safety net are sidelined.[34] Intersectional approaches push us to consider both–and hypotheses that better reflect actual human decision-making.

The size of the Latino millennial population is another excellent reason for scholars to unpack Latinos' diverse relationships with different government agencies and programs.[35] Recall that Latino millennials make up nearly half of the 10.1 million uninsured but eligible US Latino population; then consider the group's likelihood of racialized experiences with state bureaucracies.[36] To date, much of the research on Latino millennials has focused on their interactions with the criminal justice system, education system, or immigration enforcement system.[37] This book advances research on Latino millennials by extending a focus on their experiences with health insurance.

Perhaps the greatest benefit of an intersectional approach is its emphasis on social structures working in tandem rather than in isolation or competition. Standard social scientific approaches put structures like race, class, or gender in a hierarchy by using qualitative or quantitative metrics to determine which is more or less important in predicting an outcome. In practice, this frequently results in the researcher choosing their favorite social category as the sole focus of their research. These tendencies have contributed to the balkanization of subfields, such that social structures like gender or sexuality are treated as their own separate fields of study rather than integral considerations in health policy research. The resulting errors and misspecifications can lead scholars to exclude certain social structures from their analysis, whether because they falsely presume them irrelevant or consider them other scholars' domain.

Intersectional analysis aims to articulate contextually specific connections among social structures. No particular structure is privileged, because multiple structures are at work in all places, situations, and interactions. Studying these convergences helps by broadening the possibilities we see for devising new interventions to achieve long-standing goals. In this case, that means thinking beyond ways to change Latino individuals' behavior to consider needed changes to the policies, government agencies, and nonprofit organizations shaping Latino communities. For example, health policymakers often describe Latinos as needing increased health literacy, defined as "the degree to which individuals have the capacity to obtain, process, and understand basic health information and services needed to make appropriate health decisions."[38] The concept of health literacy, however, suggests that there is only one correct way of interpreting health care information, pathologizes alternative forms of knowledge about health insurance, and oversimplifies the many ways people acquire knowledge about health care. When an uninsured Latina refuses to apply for Medicaid, in other words, her decision may be misunderstood as an example of "health illiteracy."

An intersectional approach, on the other hand, largely "trusts" individuals' varied responses to policies, institutions, and organizations and seeks to change the latter. In this view, improving Latino health insurance coverage requires that we investigate how social structures produce various forms of knowledge—including knowledge about the state agencies with which they interact—that uninsured Latinos learn, share, and draw on when seeking (or not seeking) care. This facet of intersectionality builds on a growing body of research urging us to abandon deficit frameworks in the study of health in minority communities. For example, Laurence Ralph's ethnography of the violence-plagued west side of Chicago uncovers how residents' behaviors may be characterized as symptomatic of mental illness when, in fact, they are forms of caring for neighbors.[39] Similarly, sociologist Janet Shim's notion of "cultural health capital" emphasizes the interactional styles present in patient–doctor interactions rather than the traits of individual patients in producing uneven outcomes.[40] Capturing what is called policy learning, researchers can tap into the ways institutions, interactions, and personal networks shape knowledge accumulation among uninsured Latinos, reformulating that cultivated knowledge as a community asset on which

institutional support can be built and obviating the idea that certain behaviors indicate individual mental deficits in need of cognitive—often
criminalizing—repair.

It can be difficult to reconcile this approach with policymaking and a
philanthropic world increasingly dominated by positivist performance
metrics, statistical evaluation, and reductive and frequently biased actu-
arial risk analysis.[41] Nevertheless, by providing an alternative language
to discover and describe the structural configurations shaping Latino
health insurance enrollment, this book provides ways for advocates, organizers, and community leaders to bring intersectional thinking into
policy and philanthropic domains. One size simply can't fit all no matter how often pathologized Latino communities have been diagnosed as
desperately needing one "cure" or another.

Looking to find and dismantle the interconnected social structures
that harm uninsured Latinos, I describe, for instance, the powerful
configuration produced by the interactions between this country's systems of criminal punishment and health care. Re-centering our policy
imagination on institutional transformation is uncomfortable and it
goes against the grain of neoliberal thinking. It can be overwhelming
to consider, let alone undertake the long-term work needed to upend
institutional sources of suffering, injustice, and inequality. A policymak-
er's election cycle or a foundation's annual funding cycle is insufficient
for the ambitious structural interventions derived from intersectional
thinking. Moreover, an intersectional approach to policymaking and
philanthropic work might also help ameliorate what many call "oppression Olympics," or the unhealthy competition among different identity-
based organizations competing for grants or funding to assist Latinos
and other marginalized groups.[42]

Plan for the Book

The book proceeds with five substantive chapters addressing the four
social structures my respondents navigated as they considered health

insurance enrollment (the third, patriarchal family structures and gendered health outcomes, spans two chapters) and a conclusion. In chapter 1, I describe how the criminalization of the uninsured constrains health insurance enrollment. Uninsured participants' contacts with the criminal justice system and the specter of its hyper-surveillance shaped their perceptions and reactions to ACA outreach efforts, especially after a conviction. Intersectional analysis exposes several gross injustices produced by the intersecting structures of health care and criminal punishment.

In chapter 2, I highlight how the interlocking social structures of race and bureaucracy affected Latinos' perceptions of the health care safety net and their desire to seek insurance through the ACA, for better and for worse. Positive interactions with health care bureaucracies can go a long way toward making uninsured Latinos feel more comfortable with applying for Medicaid while enduring long waits and rude, racialized treatment can produce a far broader avoidance of state-sponsored social safety nets.

Chapter 3 turns to the contributing role of families and their patriarchal obligations in Latinas' lack of health insurance coverage. With men viewed as "natural" heads of household and primary breadwinners, Latina women described an understanding and expectation that they would sacrifice their own needs and desires in service of men. The overlapping structures of gender, family, and the health care safety net compounded barriers to health insurance coverage for this portion of my sample.

In chapter 4, I continue the focus on families, attending to the gendered distribution of family assistance that facilitates access to health insurance differently for Latino men and women. Stories in this chapter reveal the ways Latinas in patriarchal family structures subvert gendered constraints to enroll in health insurance, and others underscore the importance of family job referral networks and family health insurance plans for uninsured Latino men.

Finally, in chapter 5, I illuminate the mundane yet powerful role of college classmate referral networks in helping Latino millennials acquire health insurance. The interlocking structures of classmate networks and past health care experiences shaped how many young uninsured Latinos navigated the opportunities opened by the ACA: where respondents were initially wary about enrollment due to negative past experiences with the health care system or safety net, the policy knowledge transmitted through campus connections was particularly key in encouraging their insurance uptake.

In the conclusion, I describe the book's contributions to the study of Latino health insurance coverage, offering ideas and avenues for interventions that could actually shift social structures, weaken constraints, and foster flourishing communities.

1

How the Uninsured Are Criminalized

What would you do for the ability to breathe? This is a difficult question particularly for low-income uninsured asthmatics. The average cost of an asthma inhaler in the United States falls between $100 and $250.[1] For an Illinois citizen living in poverty (earning $1,387 or less each month), purchasing an inhaler can easily consume 10% of a month's income. The bravest might tolerate the pain and fear of an asthma attack and hope symptoms subside. If they fail, they can call 911 for an ambulance but then incur thousands of dollars of medical bills. Alternatively, they can drive or take a taxi to the county hospital emergency room, with its long waits and exorbitant medical bills. Too often, the uninsured pay through debt, physical pain, or both.

Finding those choices untenable, many low-income uninsured Latinos carve out a third path, resorting to the informal economy as a means of generating extra income (to pay for more traditional care, medications, and equipment) or acquiring health care and medications through unofficial channels. Activities can range from petty theft to the illicit purchase of prescription medications. Of course, there is no special category or mitigation in the US criminal code for health care–motivated crimes. Robbing, stealing, and buying drugs bring the risk of arrest, imprisonment, increased surveillance, and the permanent mark of a criminal record, which impedes offenders from employment upon release and even access to much-needed social safety nets.

Criminal justice and health care are, in this country, intersecting structures.[2] Too often, the study of Latinos' interactions with either are studied in isolation or placed in a hierarchy based on their predictive power.[3] In this chapter, stories drawn from my longitudinal ethnography of two individuals reveal that these interlocking structures produce gross injustices that constrain health insurance enrollment for racialized low-income people, adding vulnerabilities to vulnerabilities.

In many ways, the full extent of the criminalization of uninsurance is hidden. Health care–motivated crimes are not categorized in our legal system, which treats petty theft as petty theft, period. This makes it virtually impossible to measure the scale at which individuals have been imprisoned for health care–motivated crimes. As traumatic as arrest and imprisonment may be, the criminal justice system's most powerful constraint comes after formal punishment. The mark of a criminal record is less like a dot on your hand and more like being dyed bright green, head to toe: it affects *everything*, including your ability to get a job, let alone the kind of job that provides health insurance access.[4]

An individual's arrests and convictions—even just a so-called contact with police—train the hyper-surveillance of law enforcement more intently on them.[5] Thus, when Affordable Care Act (ACA) outreach workers and health navigators approach uninsured ex-offenders, they are often met with understandable skepticism, distrust, and concern. To eventually help with insurance enrollment, these frontline bureaucrats must first cultivate and communicate patience, understanding, and empathy.

Both respondents highlighted in this chapter's intersectional analysis, Nick and Lynette, have been convicted of and served time for crimes motivated by the need for health care. The grossest injustice of that nexus may be that they each described gaining easy and free access to health care *while in prison*.[6] Scholars have described this medicalization of the criminal justice system, noting that health care, rather than punishment, can, perversely, be used to maintain social control in prisons even as health care infrastructure in low-income minority neighborhoods crumbles.[7] These stories are what happens when these structures intersect—and what happens to the person who finds themselves at that difficult nexus. It criminalizes the uninsured, medicalizes them upon entry into the prison system, and then locks them out of employment upon reentry. Policymakers and changemakers must conceive of their advocacy for criminal record expungement as a health insurance issue and advocacy for expanded health insurance and access as a criminal justice issue.

Nick Rodriguez

Nick's asthma made him sound like a broken ventilator. It struck as we drove south on Pulaski Road, crossing over Chicago's sanitary and ship canal on our way to a movie theater. With the downtown skyline visible in the distance, I asked Nick, in the passenger seat, "When you breathe like that, what are you feeling?"

Catching his breath, Nick panted, "Like I'm breathing through a straw."

Nick pulled a green inhaler from his pocket, gave it a good shake, and inhaled a puff. His crackled breathing only slightly subsided. The inhalers he purchased out of pocket from a neighborhood drug dealer for $20 were losing effectiveness. We ditched our movie plans because Nick feared the heavily air-conditioned theater would worsen his asthma and, instead, ate lunch at a buffet in Chinatown. Nick walked gingerly from the parking lot to the restaurant.

Uninsured and 28 years old, Nick had contracted asthma in his early 20s. When his first asthma attack struck, he visited the Cook County emergency room. It was his first, and extremely expensive, introduction to the public health care safety net. He learned that each emergency room visit triggered a $6,000 bill. He learned that each asthma inhaler cost at least $100. And he learned the state could do little to help him pay these enormous bills.

Nick couldn't really turn to family for help. The youngest of three kids, Nick was largely raised by his older sister after their young Mexican American parents divorced. Their mother left the family and remarried. Their father died of cancer in 2011. And Nick's brother, a Latin King gang member, was serving a 20-year prison sentence. Now, only his older sister, Stacy, and his girlfriend, Karen, were in his life.

Living with asthma and without inhalers made it difficult for Nick to hold down a job. He finished high school but never attended college, and he tended to hop from job to job—he'd worked for Amtrak, at an air-conditioning repair company, and as an usher at the United Center where the Chicago Bulls and Blackhawks play. Developing asthma and suffering its oxygen deprivation slowed his body and mind, making Nick late to work or unable to complete basic tasks. He'd get fired after one too many screwups and then go look for another sure to be temporary job.

Employed or unemployed, Nick was uninsured, and he needed inhalers. The prospect of dying from an asthma attack haunted him. A friend referred him to a neighborhood drug dealer, and when he had cash, Nick bought the inhalers that way. When he didn't have cash, his asthma attacks sent him, begrudgingly, to the nearest hospital emergency room where he could receive care but go further into debt.

As his fear of death rose with each new asthma attack, Nick learned to prefer emergency rooms in private hospitals over the ER of his county. That first trip to Cook County had been dreadful; thus, when he saw his sister wait just 15 minutes to see a doctor in a private hospital's ER, he swore he would never go to "County" again: "I'll die in the waiting room!" He insisted, "I'd rather go into more debt than die waiting at County."

In 2013 alone, Nick had six visits to the private hospital's emergency room. That meant $60,000 in new debt, right off the top. When an ER doctor referred Nick to a pulmonologist (lung specialist), Nick borrowed $300 for the visit from his sister. Although the mold and allergy tests came back negative, the pulmonologist wanted Nick to come back in, but he simply couldn't afford it.

Uninsured and unemployed, fearing death more than his $60,000 in medical debt (but not necessarily by much), Nick was desperate. He needed money and inhalers. As a result, Nick became more deeply involved in the informal economy.

* * *

"Have you heard of Gypsies?" Nick asked me. I had.

"Do you know what they're known for?" I did not.

"Stealing."

Jobless, Nick depended on his girlfriend Karen for housing and a man he called "Ice Box" for generating income. Tall and muscular, Ice Box seemed ethnically ambiguous to strangers, but his skin tone was dark enough that he passed for Latino. Nick, who'd known Ice Box since high school, believed he was of Romani descent (hence his reference to Gypsies). The small crew Ice Box led specialized in high-end car and retail theft, as well as selling these stolen goods to a network of buyers.

In dire need of money, Nick joined Ice Box's crew. Quickly, he told me, he was only there to shoplift: "I'll never do cars," Nick said, "if you get caught, you're looking 6 to 30 years" in prison. Ice Box conferred the tricks of shoplifting in retail stores: Dress like a business professional, nice pants and a button-down shirt. Make eye contact with the employees; otherwise, you look nervous. If something feels "off," walk away. And don't sell stolen goods to friends. Instead, Ice Box referred Nick to his network of buyers in exchange for an undisclosed portion of his sales, and Nick became intimately familiar with Chicago's public transit as he traveled to drop off merchandise for customers in neighborhoods both rich and poor.

Nick started with iPads, swiped from Target displays, then moved to higher-end retailers as he gained experience and skill.

"I'm coming up on Macy's downtown," said Nick as we stopped for burritos in Little Village, "like $10,000 worth of merchandise."

"Really?" I asked skeptically.

As he chewed his food, Nick pulled out his phone and showed me his Facebook account. He scrolled through dozens of photos of himself, posing with his girlfriend and all sorts of merchandise. Purses, sunglasses, high-end high heels from coveted brands like Michael Kors, even luxury purses. Nick took special pride in the Louis Vuitton theft: "It was a $1,000 purse I sold for $8,000."

Nick's shoplifting and resale income went toward paying down his medical debt and buying asthma inhalers. Trial and error had taught him to prefer Symbicort's and Advair's versions, which contained both a corticosteroid and a bronchodilator but had their own luxury price tags: at a CVS Pharmacy, paying retail cost between $310 and $527 for 120 doses. The neighborhood drug dealer got them to Nick for $25.

It wasn't very long before Nick's shoplifting gig had earned him more money and luxury goods than he anticipated. He gifted items he could not sell to his girlfriend Karen, who knew about his illicit activities. After a few months, Karen even accompanied Nick on some of his shoplifting excursions. Eventually, Nick bought a diamond ring and proposed to Karen. She said yes.

Everything changed when Nick and Karen decided to steal iPads from a Target store. A customer spotted Nick breaking the lock on the display case and notified security who immediately called the police. Nick and Karen were confronted and arrested just as they were about to leave. They were both charged with misdemeanor retail theft, but because neither had any prior criminal record, they were spared prison time. Each was fined $3,000 each and given two months' probation. Terrified, Karen demanded Nick quit shoplifting—a second arrest would land him in prison. Nick promised: no more stealing.

But Nick's promise was unsustainable. With no savings and no income, he could not afford inhalers, let alone their $3,000 fines and payments on his tens of thousands of dollars in medical debt. After two months without getting a job offer, Nick shoplifted again and got arrested again. Like before, a customer saw Nick stealing; this time, the customer was an off-duty police officer.

Nick remembered, "This guy was dressed in regular clothes, but came up to me, pulled out his badge, and told me I was under arrest." Stacy, his older sister, bailed him out of jail. Karen, however, called off their engagement and broke up with Nick. "She told me I lied to her and that she could never trust me again," he told me. Despite the breakup, Nick and Karen remained friends.

Nick pled guilty to felony retail theft (the purse he attempted to steal was valued at more than $300). Since it was his second offense, he received a three-year prison sentence with the possibility of early release for good behavior. Nick's time in one of downstate Illinois's prisons, he said, was less difficult than he anticipated. Ironically, Nick claimed he got some of the best medical treatment he's ever had for his asthma when he was locked up.

"Did you have asthma attacks in jail?" I asked.

"Yeah, but I had treatment there. I was given inhalers and pills. Lots of pills." Along with inhalers, prison health workers put Nick on a cocktail of sedatives like hydroxyzine, Klonopin, and Prozac (typically used for treating anxiety, they can prevent asthma attacks). Nick never needed emergency care the whole time he was in prison.[8]

The stories Nick told me about his prison experience illustrated several dimensions of the interlocking structures of health care and criminal justice. The criminalization of uninsurance was certainly evident, as Nick was imprisoned for a crime committed in response to inadequate health care (he had returned to shoplifting after being unable to get a "real" job after his first brush with the law). So, too, is the medicalization of the criminal justice system: prison was the first time Nick, who lived with a life-threatening condition and frequent flare-ups, had easy, reliable, and ongoing access to proper health care.[9]

We can't know what Nick's adult life might have looked like if he'd had access to health care when his asthma first developed. What we do know is that the health system is set up so that it punishes the uninsured (first with enormous bills and hounding debt collectors and then through individuals' responses to managing those costs) and, at the same time, it turns a profit from providing contracted health care for imprisoned populations.

Nick's experience after prison, in reentry, revealed another cascade of consequences stemming from the interstices of the health care and criminal justice systems. He was now trapped in a state of perpetual economic crisis. He'd lost Karen (and, with her, his housing—hard to replace for a convicted felon when landlords conduct background checks and for a debtor, since they check credit histories, too). His criminal record, and the fact that it was for repeated retail theft, virtually eliminated his formal labor market prospects and any hope of employer-provided health insurance.[10] With only Stacy and Ice Box remaining in his social network, Nick found the informal economy tempting, but he was determined to get back on his feet and win back Karen. He just had to stay alive.

* * *

In January 2015, Nick was released after one year for good behavior and moved in with his sister Stacy (a car salesperson) and her husband Jack (an electrician). Fresh out of prison and with little money, Nick depended on them for basic needs, including temporary housing. No longer shoplifting to buy inhalers but unable to secure employment, Nick worked as a day laborer, earning a few hundred dollars per week, and went to the emergency room when asthma attacks inevitably left him breathless.[11]

As Nick struggled, Medicaid expansion was underway in Illinois. Because he was now eligible, I asked whether he was going to try to get health insurance through the ACA.

"Right now, I want to see what happens. If I hear it's helping people, then I'll get it," he responded. It was a far cry from his attitude when we first met: rather than talk about his fear that he'd die in a Cook County Hospital waiting room, he'd become open to interacting with the county's health care system.

It turned out one positive, if counterintuitive, aspect of Nick's time in prison was that it made him more comfortable seeking public assistance. He'd begun to think government might actually be able to provide some help.

The ACA really entered his consciousness on the streets of Little Village, where the policy's implementation "navigators" fanned out, knocking on doors and passing out flyers, trying to identify and enroll

uninsured individuals. It was an effort going on in low-income neighborhoods around the country.

"A woman approached me, asking if I had health insurance," Nick
recalled. "She told me I should get the Obamacare, that it would get me
my asthma medication and even help pay my medical debt."

"Did you give her your information?" I asked.

"I did, but when she called me back, she called from her cell phone,
which I thought was weird. Aren't they supposed to call you from an office? . . . Seems shady to me."

Nick never followed up, because his experience with Ice Box made
him aware of identity theft scams, which negatively shaped his perceptions of ACA outreach workers.

Months later, however, Nick called me to share that he "got on Obamacare." After a severe asthma attack, an emergency room administrator
had come to his bedside and convinced him to apply for Medicaid. "The
lady just told me I should sign up, and I was like, 'OK. Sign me up.' They
walked me over to a clinic inside the hospital, asked me a few questions,
I signed some papers, and that was it."

It was, for Nick, far more comfortable applying for health insurance
on the recommendation of an administrator in a hospital emergency
department than with the navigator he met on the street. Their pleasant
and helpful interaction fit with his positive experience with prison medical personnel, too, and so his time in prison made him more comfortable using the health care safety net on the outside.

This interaction helped enroll Nick in Medicaid and provided him
with a prescription for multiple inhalers that now only cost him $7.

Medicaid enrollment fundamentally improved Nick's life. His new
inhaler prescriptions cost just $7 out of pocket, so, although he was still
without a job, he didn't have to choose between shoplifting and risking
jail or going without preventive care and risking death. The next time
we hung out, Nick was carrying three inhalers at all times: the blue one
was for minor asthma symptoms, yellow for more severe, and red for
worst-case scenarios. The red inhaler contained Prednisone, a power-

ful, brand-name steroid that, by reducing inflammation, opens airways almost like a muscle relaxer for the lungs. If and when Nick needed to refill these prescriptions, he visited his new primary care physician at a Cook County clinic just a few blocks from where he lived with Stacy and Jack.

When it came to Stacy and Jack, Medicaid couldn't help. The longer Nick went without a job, the more Stacy resented him. She wasn't willing to provide for all her brother's needs in perpetuity, but no matter how many applications Nick put in, his criminal record was still locking him out of a job. When Nick didn't come home some nights, Stacy wondered if he was out stealing (or worse). "When we go to the store, I would tell [Nick]," said Stacy to me as we spoke at a coffee shop, "'Please don't steal anything.' Jack refuses to go anywhere with him, because if he gets caught they would arrest Jack, too." She bought her brother an iPhone, and when he "lost it," she suspected he sold it for cash. And she remained touchy that Nick had never thanked her or her husband for bailing him out both times he got arrested.

To convince Nick to spend more time at home, Stacy bought him a puppy he named "Champion." The little Yorkie–Chihuahua mix raised his spirits, and Nick constantly posted selfies with Champion to Facebook. Things took a turn when Nick, whose red inhaler had run out, had to go to the ER with severe asthma symptoms. On his way, he asked Ice Box to watch Champion. Days later, one of Nick's neighbors found Champion with two broken legs. The puppy had run off when Ice Box left his door open.

Nick called me, infuriated, from the animal hospital. He wondered if the cops might investigate, insisting, "I want to know who did this. He's the only thing I got!" Stacy didn't hesitate to lend Nick the $500 to pay for the vet—she knew how much the dog meant to him—and Nick gratefully told her Champion's recovery would take several weeks.

Four weeks later, it was Stacy calling my cell phone, livid. "I went to check on Champion, and the vet told me they had already given him away for adoption!" I was horrified, and Stacy kept yelling.

"No! You don't understand! The vet told us that Nick didn't pay for any of the dog's medical care! That's why they gave the dog away!" Nick had left the dog at the animal hospital, pocketed Stacy's $500, and disappeared. It was my biggest clue that Nick was beginning to use exploitation to make ends meet.

Communicating with me over Facebook audio (a feature allowing for free phone calls through any internet connection), Nick later admitted to pocketing the money but claimed he didn't know the vet would give Champion away. Either way, he didn't have much time to be upset about the dog, he explained, since Stacy and Jack kicked him out. He had piled all his belongings into an old car, on loan from Ice Box, and driven off. On nights he couldn't talk a friend into letting him crash at their house, he slept in his car, parking at fast-food restaurants or in parks.

By this time, ex-fiance Karen was dating someone new. She and Nick talked occasionally through Facebook audio, although she had a program that blocked Nick from calling her. She maintained contact with Nick on her terms. After unsuccessfully "courting" Karen and beginning to wear out his welcome on friends' couches, Nick created an online dating profile. He used his old photos, posed with the luxury merchandise he had stolen, in order to get dates and get someone like Ice Box to let him shower and borrow clothes beforehand. Through the course of an evening's flirtations, Nick deceived his dates into believing he was terminally ill, with only a year to live. When they hooked up, as seemed to happen regularly, Nick convinced these women to either lend him money or let him spend the night.[12] He'd become a hustler.

At least two or three times a month, Nick called me to pick him up, usually from a different address each time, and take him to his car. I'd be driving, and Nick would pull out cash, bags of clothes, and cell phones. He'd dangle the keys to cars his dates let him borrow.

Hustling women on dating websites enabled Nick to resolve his housing crisis; he was scamming just enough money to rent a $350/month room in a house with one of Ice Box's acquaintances. Still, estranged from his remaining family, Nick was feeling socially isolated and depressed. Neither

Medicaid nor a string of lucrative hookups could help there. On Thanksgiving, he wore down Stacy, and she said he could come to her house for dinner. Fearing this was another hustle, however, she drew the line at picking him up. "Jack told me to stop babying him," Stacy explained to me, "that he can get here if he wants." Buses and trains ran less frequently on Thanksgiving, and Nick said he worried waiting outside in the cold weather might trigger his asthma. Having lost trust with his last remaining family contacts, Nick spent Thanksgiving alone in his rented room.

* * *

Nick became untraceable for a few months. Without stable housing, internet access, or a phone number, he seemed like a ghost until, one morning, he posted a photo on Facebook with a status update: "at the hospital again."

I immediately messaged Nick on Facebook messenger and learned he had been up all night coughing and, sensing a serious asthma attack coming, he skipped 911 and rode two trains before walking the last half-mile to the St. Peter's Hospital emergency room.

The following day, I picked Nick up and gave him a ride to the southwest suburb where he was now renting a room. On the drive, Nick shared that, by his reckoning, this was at least his sixth visit to St. Peter's ("one of the best hospitals," he noted) in the last three months. He wasn't, at least, going into debt because of his Medicaid coverage. When Nick added that he had stopped seeing his primary care physician, I pointed out, "There has to be a better way to manage your asthma."

After telling him, "It seems like all they do for you in the ER is hook you up to a breathing machine and give you Prednisone," I asked, "Have you ever thought about getting a small oxygen machine to keep with you at home? So, you don't have to go to the ER so often?"

"I applied for an oxygen tank, but I don't qualify for that!" Nick claimed. "I asked them, 'Do I need to die in order for me to qualify?'" At this point, we were interrupted by Nick's phone ringing (so he *did* have one, I realized).

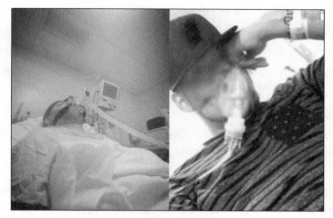

FIGURE 1.1. Photos Nick posted on his Facebook Profile.
Source: Robert Vargas.

"Hey, baby," Nick answered. "I'm still feeling pretty bad." A minute passed before he continued, "OK, I'll see you soon. Thanks, baby."

"Who was that?" I asked when the call ended.

"This girl I'm dating. Can you drop me off at her address?"

"Yeah, sure." I mentally mapped the fastest route to the woman's address and then asked directly, "Do the women you date help you out when you're in the emergency room?"

"Yeah, they do!" he chattered. "They give me a ride home. Sometimes, I have to be careful when I post a photo of myself online." This, I learned, was because Nick maintained separate social media accounts so that he could date several women simultaneously and try to keep them from learning about each other.

A few days later, I befriended Nick's various social media accounts and saw dozens of photos he'd posted of himself at the St. Peter's emergency room, timestamped July 2, July 31, September 14, October 11, November 5, and now December 13. He had message threads going with each of the women he was dating during each visit.

Locked out of employment because of his criminal record, Nick was using ER selfies to elicit sympathy and financial support across his various online profiles. The photos showed him, often wearing a breathing mask, lying in bed or sitting on a chair, and his status updates were primed for pity (see figure 2.2). In response, one or more of the women he was dating would respond by offering social or financial support, sending their Facebook messages to one account or another, never knowing about the hustle or the other women caring for him.

"One of my girlfriends visited me at the emergency room," Nick boasted with no remorse. "She said she saw on Facebook that I was in the emergency room. A few hours later she just showed up. When she came she brought drinks, candies, and some cash. She gives me hugs and kisses me. She's a lot like Karen. I like her a lot because of that." Having burned through all his family and friendship networks, Nick resorted to using the emergency room as part of his hustle to survive. This form of exploitation, of course, threatened to burn his new social ties as fast as he made them.

The constraints, injustices, and perverse incentives produced by the interlocking structures of health care and criminal justice continued to unfold over my years shadowing Nick. While the state provided free and easy access to inhalers when Nick was in prison, it also impeded his employment prospects on release. Nick's survival strategy involved using Medicaid and the emergency room to manage his illness and the exploitation of romantic partners to address his financial and emotional needs. These were the consequences of a system that criminalizes the uninsured and one criminalized individual's reliance on gendered and sexualized forms of hustling to survive after costly encounters with emergency health care and the criminal justice apparatus. Nick's behavior simultaneously reveals the injustices afflicted by interlocking social structures and how men redirect injustices overwhelmingly onto women when struggling to survive.[13]

* * *

In the final months of my research, Nick eventually found an "off the books" job with a moving company. He didn't schlep boxes, however:

bilingual, Nick handled phone calls and logistics for $30 per hour cash. It involved long drives, but he was all right with that.

Only weeks into the job, Nick's boss, the owner of the moving company, was arrested for driving with a suspended license. I did some research on the Cook County criminal records database, discovering the man's long criminal history, including seven years in prison for aggravated battery and multiple citations for driving under the influence of alcohol. Nick was undisturbed when I brought all this to his attention: "At least I know now," he responded.

It was not clear to me what exactly Nick and his boss were moving, but the police impounded the moving truck, and, with it, a book containing the addresses and schedule for all the company's upcoming moves. Although he had an appointment with the pulmonologist recommended by the St. Peter's ER doctors, Nick declared, "I need to get to Cook County Jail and get that book."

"What are you going to do?" I asked.

"I need to get that book. I don't know how I'm going to get another job."

On the morning Nick was supposed to finally meet a lung specialist, I dropped him off instead at 26th and California: the Cook County jail.

Lynnette Meriweather

The unmistakable sound of a basketball bouncing on cement greeted me at Lynnette Meriweather's North Lawndale apartment. Lynette, a 32-year-old black woman, lived with her aunt Nora and niece Ella on the first floor of the three-story Greystone building, sandwiched between two grassy vacant lots. A wrought-iron fence supported the basketball hoop and enclosed the property with its curious front yard. My interviewee, a 32-year-old black woman, was the star player on her high school basketball team and spent many days training 10-year-old Ella on this makeshift mini court.

Lynnette, Aunt Nora, and Ella were not blood relatives, but their kinship ran deep. Lynnette never knew her father, because her mother had been his mistress. When she was 14, her mother died in a car accident, and Lynnette was foisted on an uncle. In her short tenure at his house, Lynette's uncle sexually assaulted her, so she ran away. She's lived with Aunt Nora, an older friend, ever since.

Struggling with her mental health, Lynette used basketball as her escape and managed to finish high school. Fortuitously, a promising work opportunity came her way one day on her walk home from church.

"I saw people passing out flyers for Congressman Allen," Lynnette remembered. "They asked me if I wanted a job. They'd pay me $40 a day to pass out flyers. I needed the money, so I did it." Congressman Allen was a civil rights activist turned elected official with a long record of helping provide social services and health care for his poverty-stricken and predominantly African American constituents. Over time, he took the teenager under his wing, appointing her to a job supervising youth volleyball and basketball at the neighborhood park.

State budget fluctuations necessitated Lynette's ceaseless search for odd jobs. She split the rent with Aunt Nora, cobbling together her $550 per month with off-the-books work most months but not every month. She mowed neighbors' lawns, recycled metals, and refereed sports games, earning $35 for each baseball game, $50 for basketball, and $75 for football.

It almost goes without saying that, for all her work, none of these jobs came with insurance. To get medical care for minor health issues, Lynnette depended on Dr. Singh, an Indian doctor Aunt Nora recommended. He operated a clinic in the neighborhood and saw uninsured patients on a sliding scale. Lynette told me, "I would go and talk to him whenever I had a problem." Dr. Singh "was very generous. He'd give me some medications, even when I couldn't pay, and he would sometimes let me skip paying." When Ella, then five, began having difficulty breathing, Aunt Nora took her daughter to Dr. Singh, who diagnosed her with asthma.

Ella's asthma created another avenue to make much-needed cash. Dr. Singh often gave patients larger prescriptions than needed so they could have more medication at their disposal, and when Lynette accompanied Ella to her appointments, she noticed they were taking home more asthma inhalers than the little girl needed. Lynnette wondered whether she could sell those inhalers to other neighbors in need.

* * *

In the pharmacy waiting room across the street from Dr. Singh's office, Lynnette noticed a man yelling. "What am I supposed to do when I have an asthma attack?" he demanded of the pharmacist, "Go to the emergency room every night? I can't afford that." When the man stormed out, Lynnette chased after him. She offered up one of Ella's extra inhalers for just a few dollars. The man paid and expressed deep gratitude.

With that transaction, Lynnette entered the informal economy. She started by giving her phone number to people in the pharmacy waiting room, a proactive move that caught the attention of a local drug dealer. Although he also sold prescription medications, he didn't think of Lynette as a competitor. He offered her a job.

Lynette described that the dealer "saw I was good at connecting with people, so he offered me a job helping him sell: $4 for a Xanax, $5 for an Ativan, $6 for a Percocet." Lynnette and the dealer split their profits 50/50, and within weeks, people from all over the neighborhood were coming to Lynnette for the medications they needed. It wasn't, in Lynette's telling, about getting illicit substances to people seeking a high; instead, "it was mostly senior citizens approaching me on the street or calling me asking for medicine for diabetes, blood pressure, emphysema, asthma, you name it."

In fact, one day, a young man with his arm in a sling approached Lynnette, groaning in pain asking to buy medications. "I felt something off with this guy," Lynnette recalled. "I walked away because I didn't know him."

He returned hours later, but "[she] told him no again because something just didn't feel right."

When the man approached a third time, that evening, Lynnette told me, "I should have known he was a cop, but the overwhelming feeling of wanting to help someone overcame common sense." She sold the young man a dozen Vicodin, and she was in handcuffs moments later. Three police cars stormed in, and Lynette, pinned in a corner, was arrested and charged with selling narcotics. In Illinois, that felony usually meant a 5- to 10-year prison sentence. The judge sentenced Lynnette to just three years on account of her clean record and stipulated she could be released in just over a year with good behavior.

Lynnette served her prison time at a downstate Illinois facility. She had one cellmate and was impressed with the comprehensive health care. "When you enter [prison], you see a psychiatrist, counselor, therapist, and doctor. You're in isolation until you clear medical," she seemed to marvel. For a year, Lynnette spent 21 hours of every day in her cell— "just big enough for a bunk bed and a toilet," she described, noting, as the occupant of the bottom bunk, "When my cellmate had to use the restroom, she did it right there next to me." Keeping herself sane involved reading a steady stream of letters, not only from Aunt Nora and Ella but also from the neighbors they recruited to send newsy missives full of current events and the minutiae of their daily lives. Some of her new pen pals had purchased medications from Lynnette before she got locked up.

The state released Lynnette, as promised, for good behavior after a year. She moved back in with Aunt Nora and Ella and resumed her odd jobs. She entered a romantic relationship with Paul, a quiet and shy part-time security guard who, like Lynnette, was a survivor of abuse. After a few months, Paul moved into the ground-floor apartment with Lynnette, Aunt Nora, and Ella.

Unlike Nick, Lynnette found her experience with the criminal justice system was shaping her interactions with the health care safety net in multiple ways. She was now wary of interacting with strangers, scared anyone could be an undercover law enforcement agent seeking to entrap her. In our conversations, Lynnette clearly recognized the injustice of the state criminalizing communities with inadequate health care in ways Nick hadn't. For instance, reflecting on her arrest, she said bluntly, "Everything boils down to health insurance. Where else were people going to go for their medications if they don't have health insurance? I was arrested for trying to help people. I wasn't even making that much money selling the medication."[14]

At the same time, she was resourceful and remained open to the idea of receiving health insurance from the government. When I asked whether she felt the ACA would provide her adequate coverage and care, Lynette affirmed, "Yes, I do, even though people are trying to block it. The United States is a country where you have to fight for what you want. It's like what the pastor says at church, 'The race is not given to the swift, it's given to the one who endures to the end.' You got to go out and get the information to make Obamacare work for you." To her, it seemed like the coverage she and her neighbors needed was just a matter of getting through the bureaucracy and making sure others learned how you did it.

*　*　*

Coaching Ella on their front-yard court, Lynnette squatted to demonstrate a proper defensive position. She heard her knee pop and crumpled to the ground in pain. Aunt Nora took her to the nearest hospital emergency room, but learning it would cost $250 to see a knee specialist, Lynnette decided to treat herself with ice and an Epsom salt soak at home. The pain eased after a few weeks, but a heavy limp lingered, closing off some of Lynette's various odd jobs. She gained weight and desperately needed income, but it would be seven years under Illinois law before she could apply to get her criminal record expunged, and she was running into all the same closed doors Nick had. This crisis tempted Lynnette to return to selling prescription drugs, but she was too afraid she'd end up back in prison.

During this difficult period, as Lynnette sat in a youth center gym watching Ella play basketball, an ACA health navigator conducting outreach approached:

"Hi, I'm Abe. I'm working for an organization and we're trying to sign people up for the ACA."

"Really?"

"Yes, do you have health insurance now?"

"No."

"That's OK. I can assist you with enrolling. In the end, it is completely up to you to make that final decision if you want to enroll. I can start you off to see what's out there. There's Medicaid, which is completely free public assistance. With the new Medicaid, insurance companies can no longer deny you for preexisting conditions."

Lynnette raised her eyebrows in disbelief and asked, "Really?" Putting both hands in the air and stuttering, Abe "I'm not making any promises." She interrupted him again, explaining, "But that means a lot to me because I have a leg problem right now."

Navigator Abe presented his business card and contact information, and he offered to sit down with her and, with her permission, "go through the entire application." She pointedly asked, "What's in it for you? Do you get some kind of commission?" He responded that he did not and that he worked for a nonprofit, not the government. "We're just here to give people the right information to make the best decision for themselves."

The day after Lynette met Abe, she reflected on her interaction with him. I wondered why, since she was wary of strangers since her arrest, she felt comfortable booking an appointment with him. "He didn't try to sell me," Lynnette said earnestly. "He just say, 'Once we do this it's strictly up to you, just because you talk with us and give us your information doesn't mean you have to sign up, the ultimate decision is up to you.'" It came down to the style of the navigator's approach to Lynnette. His deference distinguished him from the insistent undercover officer who had entrapped her years before. He didn't seem to want anything from her.

Days later, I accompanied Lynnette for her Medicaid application meeting with Abe. She unleashed a barrage of questions, asking whether her criminal record would prevent her from receiving medical benefits, or whether her live-in boyfriend's income would affect her eligibility. Abe answered each patiently, and the appointment lasted two hours. In the end, Lynnette had applied for Medicaid, and she was enrolled only a few weeks later.

"He was really informative," Lynnette said of the health navigator, noting that "usually when you apply for any kind of public aid, you have to stand in this long line, get there at 6:30 a.m., and nobody is going to come to talk to you." Neither a cop nor a cold, public aid bureaucrat, Abe built trust and actually helped Lynette, producing quick, concrete results.[15]

Lynnette's enrollment story reveals the power of face-to-face ACA outreach strategies in undoing the damage inflicted by the criminalization of the uninsured. For the thousands of people who have been caught in the web of the criminal justice system, learning to trust and rely on a government program for assistance is no simple feat. Navigator Abe started with listening to and answering all of Lynnette's questions, tailored his outreach strategy to meet her particular needs, and empowered Lynnette by informing her that she had the freedom to enter or exit the application process at any moment without any consequences. Ceding control of the interaction, the health navigator persuaded an occasionally system-avoidant woman to apply for and ultimately enroll in Medicaid.

* * *

In 2016, I visited Lynnette at her home to follow up one last time. She still lived with Paul, Aunt Nora, and Ella, and the basketball hoop was still there. As I waited for her on the sidewalk, I spotted a woman running toward me from the end of the block. I was surprised to realize she was calling my name—it was Lynnette.

"Sorry! I was coming from the train. Can't you see, I'm running now!" she yelled out and laughed. It turned out that enrolling in Medicaid helped Lynette get back on her feet in more ways than one.

"How has getting health insurance improved your health?" I asked.

"Well, the first thing is I sleep better," Lynnette began. "Before I would sleep but I wasn't really asleep. It was hard with the pain in my leg. But now it's a lot better. It's still a little sensitive, but I can keep up the house better, I have more energy, I can exercise, referee sports again." Lynnette was also noticeably thinner, having lost much of the weight she put on because of her knee injury.

Lynnette's experience with the ACA also gave her important policy knowledge, which she used to help her neighbors. She believed that having health insurance was an important way to shield herself from poverty and the coercive forces of the criminal justice system, and she became a sort of neighborhood evangelist, spreading information about Medicaid to neighbors (including her former prescription drug customers) and helping them apply on her computer.

One day, a neighbor named Betty knocked on Lynette's door, looking for help. Her husband, Fred, was experiencing chest pains, but he didn't have health insurance. Thinking quickly, Lynnette fired up her old dusty computer with Betty and put Aunt Nora in charge of watching over Fred. Giving Betty the exact same instructions she remembered getting from the ACA navigator, Lynnette guided her neighbor through the application and printed it out.

"Go to the hospital, take this [Medicaid application] with you, and tell them you applied online. Fred will probably be eligible because he is not working."

"Are you sure?" Betty asked.

"Yes, I'm sure," Lynnette answered.

Hours later, Fred was already in the hospital when he experienced a mild heart attack. He survived, and because Lynnette had used her knowledge to quickly help him apply for Medicaid, he did not have to pay for his care—in that hospital visit or any of his subsequent care. Just as Lynnette had figured back when she was uninsured, it was all about learning how to overcome the bureaucratic hurdles. And she made sure to help others over the barricades.

Decriminalizing the Uninsured

Criminalization traps the uninsured in a cycle of perpetual crisis. They work to stabilize their lives with the tools at hand, and, as Nick's and Lynette's stories reveal, those include informal health care economies. These have been extensively studied by health care researchers focused on developing countries, yet my research suggests we need far more systematic research on the informal health care economies operating within the United States.[16] Scholars and policymakers need to look beyond individualized deficit framing, which suggests the uninsured lack "health literacy" and need to be taught the benefits of acquiring insurance and seeking medical care. Instead, I urge that we unpack the interlocking structures that place low-income uninsured people in the excruciating position of choosing among accumulating debt, committing a crime, or leaving a serious medical issue untreated. The intersectional and longitudinal ethnographic approach I apply through-out this book is beginning to reveal a path forward for those seeking to effect social change through health policy.

To start, studying the health care experiences of the formerly incarcerated is one way to illustrate the fact that health insurance decision-making takes place in the context of intersecting social structures. It's not just about medical and economic circumstances, but the seemingly impossible trade-offs people have to make to survive, as well as the experiences and informal knowledge that helps them through. For example, Nick's story revealed how gender and sexuality factored into how he used health insurance and eked out living expenses after his release from prison, whereas Lynette's decision to enroll in Medicaid stemmed from a chance encounter with a health navigator at a local community organization and later positioned her as a health resource for her neighborhood (albeit in a different capacity from her brief stint dealing prescription medications in the informal market). The social structures shaping health insurance decision-making are multiple and complex. The social science on this topic ought to be, too.

This chapter also underscores the need to think harder and more carefully about how to decriminalize informal health care economies, which economists estimate tallies up to a gross domestic product–relevant $75 to $200 billion annually.[17] This illicit market crosses race, class, gender, and age boundaries. For example, in San Francisco, narcotics officers routinely find and arrest elderly and sick individuals for selling or purchasing illicit medications, and Lynette was arrested in Chicago while selling medications to fellow neighborhood residents she believed legitimately needed them.[18] This trade is illegal, no doubt, but it's also the primary way that many uninsured Americans can survive health crises.

A useful first step toward understanding the informal health care market would be collecting data on the causes and consequences of health care–related crimes like those that put Nick and Lynette in prison. Currently, this is very difficult. For instance, the Federal Bureau of Investigation does not distinguish the illicit sale of prescription medications from the illicit sale of traditional hard drugs like cocaine and heroin; without data, health care motivated crimes remain invisible to scholars and policymakers.

Decriminalization and ending the war on drugs, one might argue, would bring a swifter end to this troubling cycle than gathering data. But to make these solutions a reality, advocates will need to marshal data to demonstrate the true characteristics and scale of health care–motivated crimes. Fruitful measures that could be enacted more quickly could involve expanding opportunities for criminal record expungement and bolstering job programs and pipelines for those undergoing reentry.

Nick's and Lynnette's stories suggest that expanding ACA enrollment among ex-offenders will also require changes in policy implementation and its public rollout. People who have been incarcerated or just had bad interactions with various criminal justice actors throughout the years may have a heightened wariness of strangers, government programs, and the possibility of getting hustled. Nick, himself a con artist, refused to enroll in Medicaid with a health navigator in his neighborhood, suspecting *she* might be a con artist, and Lynette, who had been arrested after contact with an undercover cop, grilled the health navigator who approached her at the Boys and Girls Club, trying to spot any deceit. Eventually, however, these initial contacts both resulted in Medicaid enrollments. Successful ACA outreach workers need to be trained into a hyperawareness of the multiple potential sources of wariness among their target populations, as well as the local contexts in which they work. Outreach in emergency rooms and community-based organizations appeared effective in Nick's and Lynnette's cases, and Abe, the health navigator who helped Lynnette, demonstrated that an approach that places the uninsured in control of the process, start to finish, can help even avoidant individuals feel safe, comfortable, and informed in enrollment. Lynette knew, she said, that she could discontinue the application process at any time, because Abe repeatedly made it a point to tell her so.

The case studies in this chapter are not representative of all ex-offenders, or even the population of ex-offenders in Illinois. Medicaid expansion has extended health care to thousands of often low-income people with criminal records (in the United States, 22% of the Medicaid-eligible population have a record—that's 2.86 million criminalized uninsured/potential enrollees).[19] Proponents of prisoner reentry programs view health insurance as essential to reintegration efforts, arguing that access to medical care through formal channels helps people refrain from the substance abuse or theft that landed them in prison in the first place.[20] Identifying and intervening in moments when ex-offenders face crises might help provide better access to health insurance, as well as improve overall well-being.

2

Who Deserves Health Care?

First impressions matter. As psychologists show, positive first impressions contribute to trust and social cohesion while negative first impressions can lead to fear and avoidance. Latinos' impressions of the health care system have been largely overlooked in research on health insurance enrollment. This is an important shortcoming because, for many uninsured people, the health care system's front line comes in the form of interaction with bureaucracies. Health insurance staff, public aid bureaucracies, or street-level outreach workers serve as the face-to-face representation of the health care safety net for uninsured Latinos.

Previous research has described minorities' interactions with safety net bureaucracies as sites of racialization, or processes whereby people learn what it means to be a member of their racial group.[1] Long wait times or stigmatizing interactions with staff racialize people by teaching them who does and does not deserve government assistance, who can and cannot depend on a safety net to help carry them through major crises.[2] When people of color endure documented harassment, stigmatization, and harrowing waits seeking public assistance,[3] the cumulative racializing effect becomes a chilling effect: those who feel less deserving of government assistance become less likely to apply for it, even though they are eligible.

Race scholars argue that black and Latinos' learned avoidance of public benefit programs is not accidental, it's by policy design.[4] In other words, the programs and bureaucratic processes are *meant* to keep down the numbers of people actually using public benefits rather than lowering the numbers of people who *need* them. Prior to the ACA, most major social safety net reforms eliminated rather than expanded public benefits in order to discipline low-income populations into relying less on government for survival and more on low-wage service work.[5] State governments have also shrunk food assistance programs or imposed drug tests or criminal background checks to further restrict access to public benefits.[6] The passage of the Affordable Care Act (ACA) disrupted a decades-long pattern of retrenchment in the US welfare state—drastic cutbacks and ever-more stringent eligibility rules that reflected an austere political turn toward the rhetoric of personal responsibility. These bootstrap ideologies and barriers to benefits keep the government expenditures for social support low, while frontline bureaucracy teaches would-be recipients racialized lessons that shape Latinos' shared policy intelligence.

This chapter unpacks the interlocking social structures of race and bureaucracy and how they affect uninsured Latinos' desire to seek insurance through the ACA. For example, Daniela's and Jamie's traumatic past experiences taught them to avoid public benefit programs at all cost, while Barbara and Sandra had positive experiences with the food stamps program and, as a result, felt more comfortable seeking insurance. I also share two cases of low-income uninsured whites whose experiences with bureaucracies place the racialization of the uninsured in starker relief. Their interactions with the safety net made white people feel more entitled to public benefits and confident in their abilities to successfully navigate government and bureaucracy.

In bureaucratic settings, where social structures such as race, gender, and the family intersect, individuals translate their experiences into internalized ideas about their own deservingness. Some come out of their interactions feeling supported, even empowered and motivated, to search out additional safety nets. Others leave feeling disrespected, dehumanized, and targeted in ways that amplify system avoidance. The intersectional lens applied in this chapter helps reveal the safety net, broadly defined, as deeply racialized—and it points to important lessons for outreach workers attempting to enroll uninsured Latinos under the ACA.

When Experiences with Bureaucracies Inhibit Enrollment

When we met in spring 2013, Jamie Ortiz (a 24-year-old Puerto Rican woman) worked part-time as a receptionist. She was uninsured at the time, although periodically had health insurance through her father's employer.

"My father is a truck driver," she said, "but he basically gets fired once a year. If there's not a lot of freight, they don't need him, so they just lay him off, and we lose coverage."

Jamie's private health insurance was unstable, though when she had it, she could usually count on being covered four to six months at a time. Even so, the $3,000 deductible was a shock when Jamie went to her last physical: "They charged me the full $100," Jamie recalled, "That's how I learned I have to pay the first $3,000" of each year's medical expenses. "If I knew that, I would have just tried to find a free clinic."

Indeed, a friend told her county clinics provided free testing for sexually transmitted infections, and so Jamie scheduled a visit for a day she had off work. It would affect her impression of health care for years to come.

No seats were available in the overpacked, cacophonous waiting room. Jamie's ears were flooded with the sounds of crying, laughter, cell phone conversations, printing machines, nurses and staff pacing back and forth, and the main doors sliding open and shut, open and shut. She had an appointment but waited three hours just to see the attendant—a front-desk intermediary between her and actual medical staff—who informed Jamie that, because the clinic only provided free testing on Wednesdays and not all patients show up, they had overbooked appointments.

"Yeah, we're not taking any more people today," the staff member said.

"What the hell?" Jamie said with obvious irritation. "Why couldn't you just have told me earlier?"

"Yeah, well, that's what we do sometimes," the woman said in a calm and indifferent tone. It wasn't the first time she'd delivered this news, and the receptionist quickly added that she was just a volunteer; there was nothing she could do.

Jamie returned the next week, as instructed, and was finally able to get tested. It still meant a two-and-a-half-hour wait. We debriefed after her appointment at a coffee shop in Jamie's neighborhood. She began, "Well, some of the staff were nice. I feel like people drop their preconceived perception of me when they hear me speak."

With her darker complexion and Spanish surname, and because many of the county clinic's patients were non-English speakers, Jamie believed the staff made assumptions. "Some of them talked down to me, as if I should have known this was going to be a long wait."

And that was before her test. "It upsetting because, I mean, they have volunteers who aren't really qualified."

"How do you know they're not qualified?" I asked.

"Well, I asked the lady [administering the test] where she went to nursing school and she said she didn't. Maybe she's qualified to administer an HIV test, but I wonder what can someone who is not really a nurse, not really a doctor really do for you? How can they diagnose you properly?"

"You're worried about the quality of care?" I asked.

"Yeah. I've heard stories of people who've gotten misdiagnosed and it's scary."

Her pair of visits to the county clinic effectively soured Jamie's perceptions of the ACA, another public program. When I wondered if she would try to seek health insurance now that the ACA was on the path to passage, she dismissed the idea on the basis of these experiences.

"Because, with anything that's political, it's promising a lot, but I can't say I'm sure how it's going to look once it's enacted. If it were designed for people like me to get health care, affordable health care, sure. But then, when I go, there's going to be really long lines because there's not enough people working, or the people working will be really rude. Like, I don't want to keep coming back if this is how it feels every time I'm going to the clinic. I think I would just rather not go to the doctor."

A simple preventive visit had been a distinctly racialized experience that left Jamie wary of the entire health care safety net.

"What are you going to do if you get sick?" I asked.

"I would check WebMD or Mayo Clinic [websites]."

"What about the emergency room?"

"I think I would only go if I was, like, bleeding profusely because I know emergency room rates are super-expensive. I would never go to an emergency room unless I was literally dying."

"How do you know it's expensive?"

"My younger brother was bit by a dog. He was in the ER for two hours and it was $5,000. I was 10 years old at the time, and even back then, I was like 'mental note, never go to an ER' because my mom was paying that bill off for years!"

To Jamie, the safety net was only for the direst of circumstances. Otherwise, it was best avoided altogether.

* * *

When I followed up with Jamie a year later, in 2014, she was currently covered under her father's occasional health benefits and adamant about avoiding the ACA (although she anticipated she'd lose her insurance soon). She was living with her boyfriend, and his parents helped subsidize their housing costs.

Interestingly, her new receptionist gig was in a surgeon's office. She spent a lot of time calling health insurance companies about reimbursements and informing patients of which procedures and medications their health insurance plans could and could not cover. Jamie described it as an "emotionally taxing job," filled with her concerns about the many patients who "didn't have sufficient insurance to cover the costs of procedures." On good days, Jamie helped patients learn their health insurance fully covered the procedures they needed. On bad days, she had to tell them numbers that she knew might cause financial ruin. Rather than spur her to look into ACA coverage, her interactions with health insurance at this job reinforced her fears about seeking health care and ending up with an avalanche of bills.

Another year later, in 2015, Jamie was still at the surgeon's office job and periodically covered by her father's insurance. She was now engaged to her boyfriend and told me he'd lost his ACA-extended insurance coverage under his family health plan on his 26th birthday.

Jamie was still wary, noting that her aunt and uncle had searched online for insurance and found it far beyond their budget, no matter what plan they considered, but her fiancée insisted they look around: "We looked at the prices of Obamacare online," she explained, "but those plans were basically the same price of what was being offered at his new job." In the end, Jamie refrained from acquiring health insurance through the ACA.

Daniela Salazar

Daniela Salazar, 27 years old, worked at a bar on Randolph Street, Chicago's famous West Loop row of high-end restaurants, making roughly $11,000 to $14,000 per year and living without insurance. Although she came out of her Chicago Public High School near the top of her class and enrolled at a four-year university in the city, Daniela told me, "My high school didn't prepare me for college-level courses. Being the first in my family to go to college, I didn't know how stuff worked. It was really hard balancing work, and school, and social life. I put a lot of priority into like my social life and work and not so much school." The biology major found her college workload overwhelming, dropping out during freshman year.

When we met, Daniela lived at home, with her parents and sister, in Logan Square. She was open to returning to college and maintained her aspiration to work in a biology-related field, but when she spoke about the possibility, she sounded like a battle-weary war veteran returning home—except her battles were fought against racism and sexism.

"You have to play into their system," said Daniela as she explained dropping out. "It's like if you're starting a job, you can't be yourself. You have to blend in to get ahead. In the process, you lose your culture. It separates you from your people and makes people in your racial group think less of you." This phenomenon has been described as double consciousness, a social state in which an individual with more than one social identity (in this case, as a woman who was "immensely proud of being Mexican American" and as a first-year, first-generation college student). Code-switching and trying to fit into those separate identities can make it difficult to develop a holistic sense of self.[7]

Daniela struggled with the pressure to conform to the language, culture, styles, and expectations of the predominantly white and upper-middle-class institutions she entered. Her university offered little by way of infrastructure to integrate minority students.[8] And even when she thought she was equipped with the knowledge to navigate the bureaucracies, she found it demoralizing. For instance, her high school guidance counselor helped her apply for colleges but not to handle financial aid.

"There was a problem with my financial aid, and I didn't know what was going on. I didn't even know what questions to ask. But when I went [to the financial aid office] they looked at me like I was stupid," remembered Daniela. "It's like, you have to know exactly what you're asking for; otherwise, they're very dismissive." Between the coursework and financial aid fights, Daniela decided to drop out.[9]

Daniela's brief college experience initiated a cascade of experiences that also contributed to her ACA avoidance. In particular, Daniela, who had several undocumented immigrants in her family, participated in protests against the Obama administration's increased deportations.[10]

"I feel like Obama is just a puppet who is there to make you think change is going to happen when there won't be any," she told me, disheartened by the honorary Chicagoan president's immigration actions and disregard toward the protests she joined.

"Do you think people like yourself can affect what government does?" I asked.

"I think people in positions of power can. But people at my level? No."

Due to her interactions with government and state bureaucracies thus far, Daniela had been racialized into understanding herself and other "people at my level" as second-class citizens. Dealing with the county health bureaucrats would only reinforce her sense that these systems enforce the racial inferiority of Latinos.

* * *

"Do you have any plans to look into the ACA?" I asked in October 2014.

Daniela wasted no time telling me. "No, mainly because I don't trust [the] government. I think anything they're going to be putting out is flawed."

"What makes you think that?" I followed up.

"My friend got these really strong stomach pains once and almost fainted so I took her to the county hospital. We were there sitting for hours in the emergency room! The nurses were all hanging out at the desk giggling and laughing and talking to each other, drinking their coffee, and my friend is bent over ready to pass out! I yelled at one of them, 'Are you gonna take care of her?' They came back to me laughing [telling me], 'I'm sorry, we're actually really professional.' The visit ended up costing my friend $2,300."

For my purposes, it was fascinating that Daniela spoke of the ACA and the Cook County emergency room interchangeably. For instance, when I asked if she planned to apply for Medicaid, Daniela responded, "No. With the county hospital, the staff sucks! It's like they're hiring just anybody." It didn't seem, after her friend's ER visit, like the health care safety net offered much health, care, or safety.

"Health care should be accessible for everyone," Daniela pointed out, "not just people with money." Of course, this is what the ACA was trying to help accomplish.

When I followed up with Daniela a year later, she was still uninsured. She had turned to the informal health economy, reaching out to a personal connection who, like Lynette in chapter 1, dealt in pharmaceuticals. "I know a guy who can get people access to prescription drugs," she said. "He knows I don't have health insurance, so if I need antibiotics or serious pain medicine, I can get it from him."

"How much does it cost you?" I asked.

"It depends on how much I need. At least $15. At most $60."

"How do you know you need prescription drugs?"

"I normally google my symptoms or look at WebMD. It's tough, because they list the full range of possibilities. Like if I have a skin irritation, the website lists everything from a rash to skin cancer. I tend to explore all the noncancer possibilities."

Although she spoke lightly of the range of problems she might have, Daniela's health plan took a lot of amateur physician-type labor: she researched every possible source of any illness, including how quickly it develops, its incubation period, or ways to tell if she was dealing with a bacterial or viral infection. If she believed she needed an antibacterial or antiviral drug, she would contact her informal pharmacist.

Like Jamie, Daniela never applied for insurance through the ACA during the full duration of this study.

When Bureaucracies Facilitate Enrollment

Bureaucracies and bureaucratic interactions aren't uniformly bad. In fact, in my study, two Latinas related interactions with bureaucracies that actually helped persuade them to seek insurance through the ACA. Barbara Rodriguez's experiences made her optimistic and enthusiastic to enroll in Medicaid, and Sandra Chicon's fortuitous interactions at a public aid office helped her enroll, even though she had negative past interactions with health care bureaucracies that influenced how she ultimately used Medicaid.

Sandra Chicon

"I'm going to the school of life right now," said Sandra, a 21-year-old Mexican American lesbian living in Little Village. Sandra completed high school but wasn't in college. After working 40 hours a week waiting tables at her family's restaurant and going to school from the age of 14 to 18 (her mom operated the cash register while her stepfather cooked), she needed a break. Sandra's biological father lived in Mexico (he was being deported when she was 10), and neither her mother nor stepfather completed high school. They were Catholics, and so Sandra felt alienated even though she spent so much time with her family.

"I lived in shame of my sexual orientation," she commented, because her family made her feel homosexuality was a sin. Luckily, a neighborhood youth group provided a safe space for Sandra to open up about these pressures. Housed at a nonprofit social justice organization, the youth group provided kids an education on social issues afflicting their neighborhood and provided a haven from work, family, and school pressures. At 18, Sandra accompanied the youth group on a spiritual retreat led by a Mexican indigenous leader. It was a revelatory experience.

"The retreat taught me the importance of forgiveness," Sandra described, "not only about forgiving other people, but forgiving myself for feeling ashamed of who I am. I realized I was giving so much to others, but forgot I had a responsibility to myself." She decided she needed time after graduation to rediscover herself.

It was 2013 when I first spoke with Sandra. The ACA was unrolling, and she was uninsured, but Sandra did not think the ACA would have much to offer.

"Health insurance for me is about making sure that pharmaceutical companies and doctors continue to profit," she said, "all while no healing takes place in our communities." Her mother, Sandra said, was on medications for high blood pressure, hypertension, headaches, bone aches, and ulcers. Sandra joked, "It's like she has her own little pharmacy." But none of it made her mom *healthier*: "Medications just sedate us," Sandra argued, "they don't treat the root causes."

Like many other children in immigrant families, Sandra had long served as a translator between her parents and grandparents and layers of bureaucracy and institutions of all sorts. A trip to the Cook County emergency room stood out in her memory as particularly dehumanizing. "My grandmother didn't have health insurance and she was in severe pain but we didn't know why. We took her to County and it was like, 'Whoa.' From the level of poverty to the long wait to how the staff make you feel . . ."

"What feeling?"

"Like you're not human. Like you're a number. They treated my grandmother so dismissively. I had to translate for them and tell my grandmother they thought her pain was nothing. My grandmother kept telling me to tell them she was in a lot [of] pain, and the [ER workers] were like 'no, no, no, it's nothing.'"

It is possible that the staff actually had carefully taken the woman's vitals were trying to reassure her that, although she was in pain, this was not a life-threatening situation. But much can be lost in translation, especially if communicated improperly amid the chaos of an emergency room full of misery and fear. The situation would be tough for any adult, let alone a child.

"We waited four hours for a 20-minute meeting with a doctor. They told her she had 'bone aches' and prescribed her pain medicine." Sandra stored away the experience, folding it into her knowledge of health care in general.

"When I get sick, I always ask myself, 'Is it worth it to go?'" For Sandra, the answer had always been no.

"Any plans to look into the ACA?" I asked.

"No, I plan to stay away."

"Why?"

Equating clinics with the pharmaceutical giants, she continued. "Because it's part of a bigger system, a system which has really destroyed our communities. Like, my mom is on all these medications—it's like an addiction. It's not meant to heal; it's meant to numb the pain. It just continues this cycle of control." With opioid deaths still rising, she had a point.

"Then what will you do when you get sick?" I asked.

"Well, I think about the pain, and think about whether it's really worth trying to go to the hospital. I usually wait a few hours or a few days, try home remedies, or call my friend who is a nurse practitioner for advice. But if it's absolutely unbearable, I'd have to go to County." She hadn't yet and considered herself lucky for it.

* * *

"I heard that if you didn't get health insurance, you were going to be charged a penalty," Sandra told me a year later, in 2014. "So I was like 'oh shit, let me look into it then.'" Although Sandra's perception was inaccurate (her income was too low to trigger a penalty for uninsurance, and the tax penalties were struck down by the US Supreme Court), Sandra's fear-driven motivation to inquire about the ACA was consistent with studies showing that fear of the policy's tax penalties contributed to enrollment increases in the first year of ACA implementation.[11]

Sandra found a solution by enrolling in her stepfather's health insurance plan. He was working at a construction company by then, operating a pulverizer (a heavy tool that breaks up concrete), and his employer offered insurance benefits. Not long after Sandra enrolled in his family plan, however, her stepfather developed severe arthritis in his hands. It was clearly related to his work, and the insurer wanted his employer to pay his medical bills; his employer claimed he was not entitled to worker's compensation. The stalemate put Sandra's family in a financial crisis compounded when, weeks later, Sandra was laid off from her part-time job at a day-care center due to slow business.

Uninsured again and needing to make ends meet, Sandra accompanied her stepfather to apply for unemployment benefits and food stamps at the public aid office on Cermak and Ogden Avenue. He "got food stamps right away, but he was ashamed to use them," she remembered. "One day, he asked me if I wanted to go grocery shopping with him. I thought he wanted to spend quality time with me. When it came time to pay, he gave me the link card [food stamps card] and told me to go pay. I guess he thought it was more appropriate for a woman to use it than him."

Stressed and in pain, Sandra's stepfather turned to alcohol. Home became a toxic environment full of verbal abuse. It escalated until he was pounding on Sandra's bedroom door: "My mom was in Mexico at the time, and he was drunk. He kept pounding on my door saying we need to talk."

"About what?" I wondered.

"He kept saying 'Eres mujer o hombre?' which means, are you a woman or man?"

In the year since our last interview, Sandra had begun embracing her sexual identity, defying gender norms with respect to clothing, manner of speech, and hairstyle. She had not come out to her parents, but they clearly had their suspicions. When her stepfather was drunk, he violated their informal "don't ask don't tell" policy, and she no longer felt safe. Sandra's mother understood her decision to move out.

"My mom was very upset he did that," Sandra said. "She told me I had to be somewhere where I felt comfortable being myself."

"That must have meant a lot," I commented.

"Yeah, it did." Sandra explained, "I knew [leaving home] was going to be hard for them financially, but my mom said that, in the past, she had been in abusive relationships but waited too long to leave. She stuck around and took a lot of punches, physically and emotionally. Her advice to me was just 'Go!'"

After a tearful good-bye, Sandra moved in temporarily with Erin, an older friend she had met on that spiritual retreat years before. Erin's home in Chicago's predominantly African American Woodlawn neighborhood provided Sandra a much-needed safe space, and Sandra turned to Erin for advice on managing the life changes that came with embracing a queer Latina identity.

Sandra, however, was on the verge of an economic crisis. She needed income. To help her get by, Sandra went to apply for unemployment benefits at the same public aid office she'd gone to with her stepfather. As she got started with the paperwork, the welfare bureaucrat informed Sandra she could also apply for Medicaid through Obamacare. "Why not?" Sandra asked rhetorically. "My situation is basically an economic emergency. I need all the help I can get." With help from the public aid office, Sandra was enrolled in Medicaid within weeks.

The interlocking structures of health care, public aid, sexuality, and the family all played overlapping roles in priming Sandra to accept this opportunity when it presented itself. Helping another apply for public aid introduced Sandra to the idea that the state can and, in fact, provide some assistance. Escaping her stepfather's abusive and homophobic behavior forced Sandra into financial crisis. Together, both events contributed to Sandra visiting the public aid office, leaving with food stamps and a Medicaid application.

It is important to note that the ease with which Sandra applied for and enrolled in Medicaid at the public aid office was by design. In moving to an electronic platform for all public benefit applications, the Illinois Department of Health and Family Services had purposefully retooled its website to let users apply for multiple forms of benefits at once. For example, if someone started a food stamps application, the user would be prompted that they could also apply for Medicaid and/or cash assistance. Public aid workers, in Sandra's case, did the same in person, complementing the work of the ACA navigator teams we met in chapter 1. This seemingly mundane technological and bureaucratic tweak—bundling applications for aid programs with similar eligibility requirements—proved crucial in getting Sandra on her feet.

* * *

"You still haven't *used* it?" I asked about her experience with Medicaid.

Six months passed since Sandra moved out of her parents' house. She had a job with the Chicago Park District and shared an apartment with her partner. We clutched hot coffee cups in our hands as we talked on that frigid Chicago day.

"I haven't used it," she confirmed.

"Why?" I asked.

"I just think about how much time it would take for me to go see a doctor. The hours I would lose from work. How long I would have to wait."

It turned out, Sandra's prior experience at the Cook County emergency room hadn't been pushed aside by getting Medicaid insurance. "You know, you have to take a number and wait there for three hours. And then drive all the way back home," she told me, "I'm assuming that would be the same situation."

As with emergency rooms in general, Sandra understood using Medicaid as risky and only for when "things really hit the fan." Her negative past experiences still shaped how she used her new insurance, and so she continued to rely on the informal health economy. When Sandra got sick, she got by with a combination of home remedies and connections to people selling prescription medications.

"I don't know if this is right or wrong," Sandra prefaced before revealing, "but there's a little clothing store in a nearby neighborhood that sells antibiotics from overseas. There are these little gray-colored pills for $10."

"What do you do? Go to the counter and ask?"

"Yeah. Not many people know they sell it. The store owner is a self-made entrepreneur and former gang member. He's very friendly. But yeah, if you ask for penicillin, they have it behind the counter in a desk."

An undocumented immigrant, Sandra's partner clued her into the ways she, too, could acquire medical assistance through the informal economy. (The ACA prohibited undocumented immigrants from enrolling in Medicaid or purchasing subsidized health insurance plans through the online marketplaces.[12]) But when the couple was riding bikes in a forest preserve one afternoon, Sandra was distracted and crashed into a tree. Clambering up to stand, she felt pain shoot from the big toe on her right foot right up her leg. When the swelling and pain got worse, Sandra's partner convinced her to go to the emergency room.

Now, Sandra had Medicaid and knew the visit wouldn't mean a huge medical bill. What she didn't know was that she could use it at all kinds of facilities. She believed Medicaid only covered care at overcrowded emergency rooms like Cook County. Thus, Sandra insisted on going to Saint Jerome's hospital, where she knew low-income friends and family members in her new neighborhood routinely went. "Saint Jerome is kind of the 'ghetto hospital' . . . considered the worst hospital in the South Side," she explained to me.

"Why not go somewhere else?" I asked.

"Because I don't think they would take someone like me."

Sandra's decision to visit the "ghetto" hospital came out of her past experiences with health care bureaucracies. Race scholars describe this dynamic as the consequences of structural racism, which conditioned her to believe that any insurance "people like her" could get (including her Medicaid) only covered lower-quality care at lower-quality facilities.[13] That's what the system had communicated to her through racialized and class-inflected bureaucratic interactions.

At St. Joseph's, Sandra had another poor experience: after a two-hour wait, she described, "I went in there, they took X-rays, and were like, 'Yeah, it's fractured.'" The doctors taped her foot and put her in a walking cast ("a boot"). It felt perfunctory. "If I knew it was going to be that simple, I wouldn't have gone."

An additional snafu in which Sandra's paperwork listed her as "self-pay" meant she had to "put the $900" cost of the visit on her credit card. "They told me that Medicaid could reimburse me for that cost."

"Were you reimbursed?"

"I did [get reimbursed]. I followed the instructions they gave me. It was pretty smooth. Overall, I was there for three hours, which, by our standards, is pretty good."

I mentally flagged the phrase "our standards." With those words, Sandra again identifies herself as belonging to a category of citizens seen by institutions as less deserving of assistance from the health care safety net. I understood that, with Medicaid, Sandra could have taken her broken toe to any hospital emergency room in the city—Medicaid would have reimbursed her no matter which facility she chose. The lessons she internalized from past experience had taught her instead to (1) only use the health care safety net in times of extreme crisis and (2) go to the overcrowded facilities she perceived as minority-serving.

Barbara Rodriguez

Barbara Rodriguez was born and raised on the US side of the southern border with Mexico, and she moved to Chicago at the start of high school. In our first interview, Barbara (age 24) also expressed a deep disdain for the Cook County health care system.

"It's a pain in the ass because you go in there and your brain thinks 'poor.'" Prior experience with the county health clinics had been negative: "you see people in there speaking wildly, not caring, not giving a fuck, dressed raggedy. It makes me not want to give a fuck either." In high school, Barbara had gone in suffering from a particularly bad flu and remembered the staff as impatient rather than caring: "They look annoyed all the time because there were so many people." Plus, she told me, using the county health care system meant giving up your entire day; with long waits, it was impossible to plan on making it to school or work.

Barbara had been uninsured since age 19. "When I get sick, I buy over-the-counter products. If it's really bad, I stay in bed and just sleep all day for a couple days, drink a lot of orange juice and water." So far, this self-care had worked.

Given her negative experiences with public health, I was somewhat surprised at Barbara's response to the ACA and the benefits it might bring.

"Do you trust the ACA will provide you adequate health care?" I asked.

"I'm optimistic," Barbara answered.

"What?" I said, "after all you've been through?"

"It might be like County [hospital]. It might not. But I think it will ultimately be a good thing."

"Tell me about your optimism."

"Well, some insurance is better than none. I think that's the source of my optimism. Although my experiences in the past have not always been the best, I have had access to some benefits."

Through her whole childhood and then her high school years in Chicago, Barbara shared, her family had received food stamps. As a teenager, it could be a bit embarrassing, she admitted. "I'd make sure none of my friends were at the store or working the cash register," Barbara recalled, but "sometimes we'd run into a teacher or friend from school, and I'd be like 'fuck!'" In those days, it was easier to get "busted" this way, because the food stamp payment card, called a "link card," was emblazoned with enormous capital letters: LINK. That was tough to hide and being on food stamps carried the stigma of poverty. (Today, the cards look like Visa debit cards.)

Nonetheless, Barbara vividly remembered that food stamps *helped*. "We had some rough times where we'd be low on food for a month or two. I remember being so hungry. I'd look in the pantry for a snack and see nothing. When the link card arrived in the mail, it really helped us out." With this assistance, Barbara's family could come together for home-cooked meals. The memory of gathering around the dinner table with her parents and siblings, sharing chorizo with eggs and tortillas, had never faded. "I don't think about those times often," Barbara said, "but it's in the back of my mind. I could let it make me angry, but I don't. Instead, I choose to use it as a source of pride. To me, those memories mean I've worked hard and struggled through things."

Barbara dug through her purse for a few seconds and pulled out her old LINK card. A bit faded by time, the letters LINK remained big and bold. "I keep this in my purse so that I never forget about what I've been through," she said as she looked at the card. "It makes me feel stronger . . . stronger than people who have had more privilege in their life."

I asked the young woman to expand on the lessons learned from participating in the food stamps program, and she replied emphatically, "That welfare programs can really, really, help families that do work hard and do need them. I recognize there are people who milk the system, but these welfare programs are necessary because they just aren't opportunities for everyone in society to succeed. Given the resources this country has, and how much poverty there is, it's like these programs are a way to prevent people from revolting and going crazy. It's like government throws starving people a piece of bread so they don't burn everything down."

Maybe the help, in other words, wasn't entirely benevolent, but government assistance really could make the difference in getting through difficult times. This positive experience was physically embodied in the link card she kept with her after all these years, and it canceled out (or at least balanced) the bad experiences she'd had with the social safety net as deployed at the Cook County clinic.

Another program Barbara felt good about was Medicare, the federal health insurance program for the elderly. "My dad is on Medicare," she noted, adding that he is diabetic, "but goes to private hospitals." Hopefully, she added, "So I think with Obamacare, it'll be possible to do the same." Unlike many other uninsured Latinos in this study, Barbara had seen firsthand that government insurance programs could be used at not only overcrowded county clinics but also a variety of medical providers. "When my father goes to the doctor it's a mix of people," Barbara noticed when she accompanied him. "They weren't all poor. It wasn't a long wait."

Brightly but with realism, she told me, "The system is inefficient, [government programs] can be run better, but [the ACA] is a step in the right direction. It's going to help cover more people, but not everyone. I know there is a penalty for not having insurance, which is fine if they make it affordable enough for everyone to buy."

"Do you plan on getting health insurance through the ACA?" I asked.

"If I learn it's cheap enough, yes. If it's not, then no."

* * *

Barbara, a part-time student, graduated from college at age 25 and went to live in Mexico with extended family for a year. She wanted a gap year to rest; then she would begin applying to master's programs. Still uninsured, she was fortunate to not get sick or need serious medical care while abroad. In the fall of 2015, she returned to Chicago, moved in with roommates in Logan Square, and began working three jobs. On weekdays, she worked part-time at a day-care center; on weekends, she worked at a Chuck E. Cheese restaurant; and a few days a month, she worked with a wedding planning group. None of her jobs offered health insurance, so Barbara looked into the ACA.

First, she went to the healthcare.gov website via Google. After following all the prompts and entering all her personal information, she learned she may be eligible for Medicaid. That sent her to the Illinois Medicaid application website (abe.illinois.gov), where she calculated that her combined income from three jobs still left her eligible. She applied.

When we met for coffee a month later, Barbara was visibly shaken. She launched right in: "I never realized how important health insurance is until now." I asked what happened, and she said plainly, "I got pregnant and needed an abortion."

With her Medicaid application still in process, Barbara was unsure how to get help. Ultimately, she turned back to Google, searching women's health centers in the Chicagoland area. She chose one and hurried there.

"I told them I didn't have any money," she recalled, "and they said it was fine. They were so amazing. When I sat down to wait, I looked around and thought, 'This is why it's important to have health insurance.'"

The clinic was able to provide Barbara's abortion procedure, and the staff instructed Barbara to keep her payment receipt and submit it to the state for reimbursement, since her Medicaid application was already in progress. A few forms and a few weeks later, the Illinois Department of

Health and Family services sent her full reimbursement. Even better, in her mind, was that the clinic had offered up a number of birth control options that are more reliable than the forms she had been using when she got pregnant. Specifically, the clinic recommended an intrauterine device (or IUD), which is inserted into the uterus, prevents conception, is 99% effective, and can remain in place for up to a decade (with full fertility on removal at any point). Barbara's forthcoming Medicaid coverage meant getting an IUD would be free for her, because the ACA required all plans to provide birth control coverage with no cost-sharing or out-of-pocket costs like deductibles, copays, or co-insurance.[14] A month later, her Medicaid in place, Barbara returned to the women's health clinic to get her IUD, no charge.

I mentioned to Barbara that, since women's reproductive health is a divisive political issue in the United States, some readers might find her story troubling. Could she talk about the benefits of access to reproductive care through Medicaid?

"It's been great," Barbara said, "because I'm not going to fuck up my life by having a kid I don't want. It's huge. This can seriously fuck up your life. Not just having a kid early, but having to go through the mental stress of getting an abortion. [My friend], who had an abortion, lost a semester at school. It messed her up emotionally. It messed up her life." Barbara also tied reliable birth control, safe abortion care, and reproductive health coverage to inequality: "it's also something higher-income people have access to, it's something they don't have to worry about."

Going further, she said of the IUD in particular, "It's helpful because it protects you, not just from getting pregnant, but from people or forces who will try to make you feel ashamed of yourself for getting an abortion. When you go through [an abortion], it's hard to find someone who can empathize. It's isolating, even if you have friends who have gone through it. My best friend didn't even want to tell me [about her abortion]!"

Health insurance is often thought of as financial and physical protection. Barbara's story, of needing reproductive care, in particular, demonstrated that health insurance also protects people from social and emotional harm. People who obtain abortions are more likely than others to report depression, anxiety, suicidal ideation and behaviors, and substance abuse problems.[15] But *abortions don't cause these problems.* It's the stigma and isolation attached to the interlocking social structures of the family, health care, and public aid that cause these problems. By expanding Medicaid eligibility and mandating coverage for reproductive medications and services, the ACA has helped 55 million Americans gain access to what Barbara described as a bulwark against stigma.[16] I expect that Barbara's story would be echoed by countless others.

From food stamp receipt in childhood to her father's experiences with Medicaid, Barbara had a sense that the safety net was, in fact, for people like her. Receiving reproductive health services through Medicaid and the ACA reinforced that belief. When I followed up with her a year later, in the summer of 2016, Barbara was preparing to move to Florida and start her master's degree program in economics. And she made sure that she helped her mother and siblings apply for enrollment in Medicaid.

"My family is not very tech-savvy," Barbara said. "They get most of their information through letters in the mail, and they can't read English very well." She noticed that her mother was eligible for Medicaid but had been paying out of pocket for medical care at a private practice in the neighborhood for years. "They didn't know about Medicaid. I thought somebody at the doctor's office would tell them but no, so I did it for her." As a result, Barbara's parents now have regular access to doctors. Her positive experience on Medicaid contributed to her encouraging and helping others to enroll, something she had never done before.

In contrast to other respondents in this study, Barbara's past experiences with bureaucracies were quite positive, an impression that seemed likely to continue into the future.

"Do you still carry the LINK card with you?" I asked.

"I still do. It carries the same meaning, that the older I get, the more successful I get, I remember where I came from."

Bureaucracy and Deservingness among Whites

While this book focuses on Latinos (and chapter 1 included the case of Lynette, an uninsured African American woman), I include in this chapter the experiences of two low-income, uninsured whites. These cases serve as a descriptive counterexample, demonstrating that the forces of race and bureaucracy can work to instill confidence, a sense of belonging, and a sense of entitlement in some citizens. Uninsured whites' experiences with health care bureaucracies were radically different from most Latinos', and they often ended with much more positive outcomes and attitudes toward the ACA.

When I first stepped into Sharon Kelly's Logan Square apartment, she was in the kitchen preparing a large batch of meals. After difficulties finding stable employment with her psychology degree, Sharon earned income as a yoga instructor and a caregiver for elderly persons, as well as selling healthy meals to her time-constrained yoga students. Originally from California, Sharon moved to Chicago for graduate school, where she met her husband, Peter, a freelance photographer.

The couple was hoping to have children. But Sharon, white and 30 years old, told me her slightly older husband's income was unstable, too. Freelance photographers are at the mercy of often short-term demand for their services, and full-time photography employment is scarce. With the precarious nature of their employment, it was difficult for Sharon and Peter to predict how much they would earn in a given year. Even in the best of times, their combined income ranged between $25,000 and $35,000 annually.

Chicago's increasingly stark economic inequality was also making it difficult to afford to raise a family. In 2014, Chicago moved up to eighth place in a ranking of urban inequality, with its highest-earning 5% bringing in an average annual income of $201,460, and the poorest 20%, $16,078. People with higher incomes were gentrifying the city's historically low-income and minority neighborhoods, including Logan Square, where Sharon and Peter had lived since 2007. Once a predominantly

Mexican area, Logan Square's average monthly rent had increased by an average of 11% each year since 2010.[17] Higher rents and gentrified retail led to property and retail tax increases, just as various city services were privatized. It was clear, when we first met, that Sharon and Peter would not be able to afford their apartment for much longer.

Health insurance—or, more precisely, their lack of it—was another worry keeping them from starting a family. According to the Illinois Department of Public Health, in 2016, the median cost of birthing a child in a Chicago area hospital was $7,709.[18] A small health complication or two can drive up that cost.

The implementation of the ACA in 2013 created an opportunity for Sharon to acquire health insurance, but she was skeptical about the policy's benefits. When I asked what she thought of the new program, she told me, "It's forcing me to get something I hope I'll never use." Revealing doubts about the US health care system as a whole, she continued. "I don't want to go into a health factory hospital for any reason unless it's an absolute emergency or if I'm having a kid. I don't really believe in checkups, because they are just looking for problems and not solutions."

In Sharon's opinion, America's health system was actually concerned about making money by selling medications rather than rooting out health problems through diet and exercise. A number of health scholars support Sharon's view. For example, while health care spending is astronomical in the United States ($8,000 per capita), most health outcomes are actually worse than those we see in similar developed countries.[19] From Sharon's perspective, continuing to invest in exercise and nutrition would do more to maintain her health than paying for health insurance she believed would provide little in return. Together, Peter and Sharon viewed the health care safety net as a resource of last resort.

After a series of failed attempts to secure higher paying and more stable employment, Sharon decided to learn more about the ACA, especially if she had a child. Her online searches suggested she might be eligible for Medicaid, although she refrained from applying. In her mind, even if Medicaid could cover the birth of a child, she wasn't certain where she and her husband would get the stable income to provide for that child.

When I followed up with Sharon a year later, she and her husband had moved to Boulder, Colorado. "We hated Chicago," she explained. "We did our best to make a life there, but the whole city just felt divided by extreme wealth and extreme poverty, and we were on the wrong side of the tracks. Socially, we didn't have many friends in the same position as us. Most of our friends were employed, and it felt embarrassing to talk about our hard times with people who were better off."

On a road trip to visit friends, the couple fell in love with the nature and beauty of the Rocky Mountains. Plus, "Boulder is this liberal pocket, and it's not so shameful to be lower-income there. At the very least, [moving here] allowed us to enjoy the beauty of nature every day." Again, leveraging the internet, Sharon found a new job that enabled their move to Boulder. The temporary but well-paying contract work for an event-planning agency required Sharon to travel for weeks at a time and then go unemployed for weeks at a time. Not ideal, but it meant Sharon and Peter could live anywhere with an airport nearby. They chose Boulder, where Peter transitioned into working as a painter for a property management company.

To learn more about their health insurance options in Colorado, Sharon and Peter visited "the county guy," a social worker at a health center in Boulder. "This poor guy made phone call after phone call trying to call insurance companies, representatives of the Colorado exchange, and he kept running into technical issues," Sharon recalled to me over the phone. After a few hours, the "county guy" told them the cheapest health insurance plan in Colorado would cover them both for $400 a month (after the ACA subsidy), and they would have a $6,000 deductible through Kaiser Permanente.

"It was depressing," Sharon said angrily. "It was health insurance we couldn't even afford to use with that high of a deductible." Like Jamie Ortiz, earlier, the high deductible meant paying a huge amount out of pocket each year before their insurance began to cover medical expenses. And Sharon and Peter would have to find $400 in their budget each month for the privilege.

Although Sharon and Peter were disappointed, their experiences are a marked difference from those described by the uninsured Latinos in this chapter. The "county guy" social worker not only treated Sharon and Peter with respect; he also spent hours personally calling insurance companies to help them. There wasn't even a wait to see him. Sandra, Daniela, and Jamie all felt like inconveniences and burdens on the health bureaucracies with which they interacted, whereas Sharon and Peter were made to feel like they could count on staff to go out of their way to help.

Sharon and Peter did enroll in the subsidized private plan that day, but when they received the $400 bill for the first month's premium, they decided to forego it. If it came down to it, Peter, an immigrant from Europe, suggested they could travel to his home country for far cheaper medical care—maybe they could even give birth to a child in that country. Sharon and Peter decided to remain uninsured in Boulder.

* * *

When I followed up six months later, Sharon was three months' pregnant. She and her husband still had concerns, but they were ready to be parents.

Sharon called the insurance company—the same one the county social worker had found for them—and learned that their approximate annual income combined with a child on the way made them eligible for Medicaid. In Colorado, a family of three had an eligibility cutoff of $26,813, and soon they were enrolled in a Medicaid managed care program (which provides benefits and services through contracted arrangements between state agencies and private managed care organizations like Kaiser Permanente).[20] Sharon wouldn't need to go to a county hospital but could use Kaiser facilities for her prenatal, birth, and postnatal needs.

Again, in contrast to uninsured Latinos, Sharon's conversation with the frontline insurance bureaucracy was easy, respectful, and actually helpful. The contrast was not only about race and class but also the intersection of public and private benefit administration. Low-income racial minorities disproportionately interact with public aid bureaucrats instead of the warmer, more customer service–oriented private health insurance salespeople with whom Sharon interacted.

Sharon gave birth to a healthy young boy. Her interactions with county bureaucrats in Boulder continued to yield benefits. For example, Sharon and Peter stayed in touch with the social worker who had helped them navigate the ACA. With his assistance, Sharon learned about the City of Boulder's permanently affordable homeownership program (PAHP), which allowed lower-income families to purchase homes in Boulder (where the median home price is $711,800) for a fraction of the market value. Their small rental condo was owned by a landlord who purchased it through the PAHP, but because the program requires owner occupancy, the landlord needed to sell. With the social worker's help, Sharon and Peter entered the lottery for PAHP benefits and "won." The program only required Sharon and Peter to make a $2,000 down payment to buy their condo.

"We bought a condo in one of the nicest parts of Boulder at 40% market value on a painter's salary," Sharon said happily over the phone. "It was like a dream come true." Even if Sharon and Peter's income changed, they would still own the condo (they just couldn't sell it later at market value).

Receiving both health and housing benefits radically altered Sharon's beliefs about the health care safety net. She no longer hesitated to use health care or learn more about the benefits of various government programs. Reflecting on this journey, she noted, "I was absolutely skeptical at the beginning, but [the ACA] forced me to interact with public programs. It made me realize that there are programs out there if you have the tolerance and patience to keep pursuing them. I'm glad they're out there, and I wish they were more accessible to people." In sum, Sharon said, "I think it's given me hope."

No respondent in my study had a better outcome. Sharon and Peter's race- and class-based privileges fostered a much more pleasant set of interactions with bureaucracies that culminated in housing and health security for the couple and their new child.

George Price

Few of my respondents knew more about the importance of health insurance than George Price, a 29-year-old white man who worked as a bike messenger. A self-described "optimist," George graduated from a Midwest state flagship university but preferred a life behind the wheel of a bike, zipping through traffic to deliver food and packages, rather than cooped up in a cubicle.

George was optimistic when we first spoke at a bar in Logan Square, even though the federal government was on the verge of a shutdown. Texas senator Ted Cruz was, at that moment, delivering a 21-hour-long filibuster speech aimed at repealing the ACA. "I see the best in everything. Lately there's not been much good news and lots of frustration, but I got faith that this program [the ACA] will fix some things."

George attributed this generally positive demeanor to his upbringing in Dodge, Iowa. He told me that his father, a lawyer, liked to say, "Cynicism never solved anything." Not to say they didn't worry—neither parent was thrilled with George's career choice, with its high risk of physical injury, low pay, and lack of health insurance.

"Most bike messengers work for companies as 'contractors,' not employees, so messenger companies get out of providing benefits," George explained. Although it didn't provide health insurance, George chose the higher pay he could earn joining a co-op messenger company. Typically, bike messengers earn a small percentage of each delivery ($3–$5 dollars per ride) while their delivery company pockets most of the profit. In the co-op, all five co-owners split the total revenue evenly, and so George could at least save some money in case of an injury on the job.

The cumulative physical toll was another matter. His work took a toll, and George was used to letting nagging aches and pains linger. "I've had pain in my pectoral muscle for over a year," George said. "I'm sure something is wrong with it, because it just hasn't healed." And when stricken with a severe flu, George would wait it out, getting off the road and temporarily taking over the cooperative's indoor job: dispatcher. Like other respondents, he'd heard horror stories about the Cook County Hospital ER, with fellow bike messengers cursing over 18-hour waits, and so he avoided it at all costs. In the event of a serious injury, George was resigned to the fate of an enormous medical bill should he choose the nearest private hospital emergency room over a painful wait at County.

Despite his knowledge of the inefficient county emergency care system for the uninsured, George's experience gave him hope for the ACA's implementation. Years ago, he told me, he'd had severe stomach pains that lasted a full 24 hours. "I was uninsured at the time. My girlfriend thought I might need an appendectomy, which was a very terrifying situation because, well, I didn't know what was wrong with me, and I was reluctant to see a doctor because I didn't know how much it would cost. When I told her I was getting fever and chills, she said, 'Oh, that's an infection. You need to see a doctor now!' She was very adamant, so we drove around to see what we could find. It was like three or four in the morning on a Saturday. Most clinics were closed."

After an hour in the car, the couple decided to go to the Northwestern Memorial Hospital emergency room.

"Why Northwestern?" I asked.

"It was the closest to us. I wish there was an easy way to compare the price of an emergency room visit at Northwestern compared to Rush or Swedish Covenant, but I just rolled the dice." As soon as they got into the ER, George received "a cocktail of painkillers."

"I refused them at first. because I didn't know how much they'd cost, but the nurse said this was not the time to be stoic, so I just took them. . . . I think it's easier for [nurses and doctors] to just say, 'Take this,' because they are not the ones doing the charging and collecting."

George waited three hours. After ordering an imaging test, the doctor diagnosed him with a perforated appendix. He needed emergency surgery and would go on to spend three days in the hospital, recovering and fighting off the infection.

"It was terrifying in two ways. First, had I waited any longer, I could have died. Second, the hospital bill was $28,000." George spoke with the finance office to explain his economic situation, and Northwestern Memorial lowered his bill to $21,000. George left with a large bill in hand.

Months later, George remembered, he called Northwestern to inquire about financing plans. He was pleasantly surprised: "I guess they ran my info past the state, and the state picked up the rest of the tab." Even he didn't know what changed. "I really can't explain what happened. It was a situation where I didn't care to ask questions and have them discover they made a mistake. I told them to just mail me a confirmation, and I won't ask any questions." Later, I inquired with hospital officials, hoping to learn what happened with George's bill. All I learned was that sometimes private hospitals request reimbursements from the Illinois Department of Healthcare and Family Services, and sometimes those reimbursements come through.

"It was a huge relief," George said.

Thus, when I asked, "Do you think the ACA will provide you adequate health care?" George had positive perceptions of the health care safety net. "Yeah, I think it will. I know it's had problems with the website and with Republicans trying to shut it down, but I think it has good intentions. It's trying to get more people health insurance."

"Do you plan on trying to enroll in something through the ACA?"

"Yeah, my plan is to check it out soon."

Immediately after his appendectomy, George's parents implored him to enroll in a catastrophic health insurance plan. The Blue Cross/Blue Shield plan he obtained had a $6,000 deductible, but it would cover the rest of the cost of a major health emergency.

George never ended up using it because when the ACA went into effect in 2013, it mandated that health insurance eliminate certain kinds of private health insurance plans (specifically, plans that did not cover preventative care or maternity care).[21] A few weeks before I met George, he had gotten notice that his catastrophic coverage was no longer offered. This happened all over the country, and there was a major public outcry from people who lost their coverage. But George remained unfazed.

"I feel like I can affect what government does to me," George said confidently. He ticked off a list, including his experience of getting his emergency surgery paid for and the ways he's avoided paying parking tickets and certain taxes working at the bike co-op over the years. In contrast to the sense of undeservingness described by Latino respondents, this white respondent was confident that he could avoid the bad and obtain the good when it came to government.

George's upbringing in a white middle-class professional family certainly contributed to his high expectations of receiving institutional support. Although he'd heard stories, he personally hadn't had the same kind of negative experiences with overburdened hospitals or clinics that my Latino interviewees had. And, perhaps most important, unlike Sandra, George had supportive parents who worked to help him, even if his lifestyle deviated from their hopes. These contrasting cases reveal the power of race and class in structuring the uninsured people's interactions with bureaucracies, interactions that tend to make white and more privileged individuals like George feel more deserving of public assistance.

* * *

A year and a half later, George had left Chicago. Ride-sharing companies like Uber and tailored companies like Bite Squad had moved in and dominated food delivery, shrinking the demand for bike messengers. "Bike messenger work reached its ceiling," George stated. "I started seeing all these courier companies go under and, in the process, saw lawyers involved in the process of companies merging or filing for bankruptcy. It lit a light bulb in my head." Soon, George was taking on student loans to attend law school in a small town near where he grew up in Iowa.

He planned to become a lawyer and work in the field of labor law and regulation.

Shortly after beginning his degree program, George's law school instructed him to look into the Iowa Wellness program (the state's Medicaid program). His mom referred him to a local clinic where he could apply. "The navigator at the clinic explained Obamacare in a very non-political way." George noted, "[S]he kept emphasizing the purpose of everything, saying it was meant to help me." He didn't need much convincing; his self-described optimism and past experience made him comfortable applying for Medicaid.

"I know benefits for the poor are stigmatized," George explained, "but as a law student going into debt, not working, and studying all the time, I had no problem signing up for Medicaid."

Enrolling in Iowa wellness provided George his first doctor's visit in over seven years.

"When I went in, the doctor asked what he could do for me. I said, 'Well, everything I guess.'" George learned he had high cholesterol and received a referral to an orthopedist for the pain in his pectoral muscle. "I did all of that and didn't receive a single bill." The most immediate effect of having health insurance, according to George, was the mental relief.[22]

"Even after giving up bike messenging, I always worried about seriously injuring myself playing sports or trying to remain fit. I still love cycling and do it a lot, but when I'd go on a ride, I'd think to myself, 'Should I really be mountain biking without health insurance?' But now I have peace of mind. It's so assuring and comfortable." He was unlikely to ever wait 24 hours to seek medical care for serious illness or injury in the future.

* * *

At the time of our final correspondence, George was entering his final year of law school and working as a public defender. Since we last spoke, the Iowa wellness program had experienced some hiccups. Beginning on April 1, 2016, the state privatized its Medicaid programs, putting for-profit companies in charge of managing health care networks and services for Iowa's low-income populations. And because the state legislature failed to sufficiently fund the Iowa wellness program, those companies were not receiving the state reimbursement funds necessary to provide care. The *Des Moines Register* called Iowa Medicaid's payment shortfall "catastrophic."[23] Fewer and fewer doctors were willing to accept Iowa Medicaid patients.

George described experiencing some of the Medicaid challenges firsthand. When he broke his wrist biking in rural Iowa, he visited an orthopedist who was outside of his Medicaid provider network. That part went well: "It only took 30 minutes. They took an X-ray, put me in a cast, and got me out." Six weeks later, however, it was time to get the cast removed, and none of the orthopedists who learned he was on Medicaid would return his calls. "I ended up driving 90 minutes out to the rural town where I got the cast put on," he said with some amusement. Despite these troubling situations, George remained as optimistic as ever, grateful for his ACA-acquired health insurance.

Transforming the Structures of Race and Bureaucracy

When government bureaucracies help or hinder someone during a major crisis, that experience can transform their orientation toward government programs in enduring ways. Both sides of the coin are evident in this chapter. Daniela and Jamie's cases revealed the workings of a social safety net stratified by race, class, gender, and sexuality.[24] Sociologist Herb Gans once used the moniker "war against the poor" to describe how the stigmatization of welfare recipients, teenage mothers, drug addicts, and the homeless relegates many into a social class despised by the rest of society.[25] Reading the stories of the Latinos in this chapter, it seems Gans's moniker remains true for many to this day. After interactions with the safety net leave people racialized and criminalized, they can feel unworthy or untrusting of public assistance. Too often,

Latinos described learning about the ACA only after battle-wearied by their past experiences with bureaucracies, at a point when only the fear of death would compel them into seeking care from the state. They were reluctant to apply for the benefits, and in the case they did, they avoided actually using them.

Sharon's and George's experiences offer a glimpse at how interactions with bureaucracies unfold for more privileged uninsured whites. While both earned low incomes, their middle-class upbringings and white racial status had given them a different set of expectations when interacting with bureaucracies. Remarkably, both of these white respondents intentionally refrained from visiting the overcrowded county emergency rooms and clinics disproportionately frequented by low-income uninsured people of color, yet they walked away from their interactions with health bureaucrats debt-free. Sharon even learned about how to access housing assistance in addition to health insurance. Structures of race and class can produce privileges for uninsured whites, as the bureaucrats with whom they interact go above and beyond to help.

Barbara's and Sandra's stories, however, offer a glimmer of hope for uninsured Latinos. For both, positive experiences with the food stamps program facilitated their enrollment in Medicaid. Each case demonstrated that bureaucracies *can* engage in an alternative form of racialization, a form aimed at empowering rather than disempowering people of color. Barbara, without her trusty LINK card, might have gone on to resist seeking help with her unintended pregnancy, either choosing to give birth to a child she couldn't support or turning to the informal economy or other means to obtain a risky abortion in the informal health market. Imagine if more Latinos had experiences with the public aid bureaucracies that matched hers or even George's and Sharon's; surely the result would be more Latinos feeling more comfortable and confident, more empowered to interact with public aid bureaucracies to acquire benefits.

The positive experiences more often related by my white respondents may have been a big part of saving the ACA's Medicaid expansion; these empowered individuals did not hesitate, when President Trump and Republican congressional leaders tried to torpedo the program, to voice their disapproval, and they felt entitled to be heard by the people in power.

The intersections of race and bureaucracy with class and gender powerfully produced respondents' attitudes toward the ACA and, in turn, their enrollment outcomes in these stories. George, for instance, had supportive middle-class parents to fall back on, and so he was confident even the original $21,000 appendectomy bill he received wasn't going to leave him homeless. Sandra, meanwhile, fled her low-income parents' home after experiencing homophobic violence—they would not be a safety net for her in case of emergency. As a white man, George was not subject to the same structures of government surveillance like the police or immigration enforcement that affected the lives of Latina respondents like Daniela or Barbara, nor would a reproductive health problem (like Barbara's unintended pregnancy) mean George risking stigma and isolation the way it can for women, especially low-income women. When multiple structures and multiple social identities interact, as they do in health insurance access, a full understanding requires an intersectional research approach.

3

Why Latina Women Sacrifice Their Coverage

How do relationships with family members shape health insurance access among young Latino adults? This is an important question, given a convergence of trends facing the 61% of the Latino population that are younger than 35. The labor market conditions they are entering are worse than in previous generations,[1] so although Latino millennials are increasingly completing college, they have fewer options for upward mobility or stopgap jobs that provide health insurance benefits.[2] "Waithood" is what some now call the bleak period after graduation in which young people often shuttle back and forth between jobs or postsecondary education programs.[3] The economic circumstances place young adults in awkward positions with their parents, who, among other supports, frequently continue to insure their adult children through employer-provided family health plans or help their child pay premiums. Others' relationships involve family withholding support or foregoing their individual needs in favor of a relative's. The racialized and gendered dynamics of uninsured young adults' family obligations represent an underexplored force in shaping Latinos' health insurance decision-making.

Each respondent in this chapter went uninsured for the full duration of the study, in part because of the intersectional forces at play within their families. Specifically, these respondents felt doubly constrained by their limited opportunities for upward mobility coupled with gendered and racialized family obligations. Some felt—and complied with—pressure to prioritize their parents' health and financial well-being over their own. Consequently, these respondents shouldered too much of the family's needs, but the alternative was deviating from patriarchal family norms and drawing shame and threats of estrangement.[4]

Other respondents encountered a complete withdrawal of parental support, a "tough love" effort families hoped would develop financial independence and personal responsibility. This parenting strategy is akin to what Annette Lareau described as "natural growth" parenting, in which parents give children high degrees of independence and interact primarily through issuing directives or orders. Ultimately, these withdrawals of parental support were not effective lessons. They simply inhibited the respondents' access to health insurance.

I close this chapter with an uninsured white male in my study. His family obligations weren't the constraint; this respondent rejected insurance for the duration of this study due first to his luck in never needing much medical care in the past and later due to the influence of his politically conservative extended family.

"No One Was Going to Take Him In"

It was 4 a.m., and Tomas Leandro was struggling to stay awake at the wheel. Tomas, a 28-year-old Mexican American, worked at a Ford plant near the Illinois–Indiana border. It was a two-hour commute each way from his brother's apartment in Chicago's west suburbs, assuming there was traffic (and there was always traffic). "The hum of the engine puts you to sleep," Tomas recalled. He swerved, and a Chicago police officer pulled him over. Tomas remembered their exchange vividly:

"You been drinking?" the officer asked, leaning forward to take a big whiff, searching for the scent of alcohol or drugs.

"No," said Tomas.

"Where are you coming from?"

"Work. The Ford plant on the southeast side," Tomas answered.

"Oh yeah? My uncle works there. You're new to the night shift, aren't you?" the officer asked like he understood.

"Yeah," said Tomas.

"Listen, take care of what you need to take care of. Force your body to adapt. If I see you swerving like that again, I'm going to arrest you and suspend your license," the officer warned.

Tomas agreed and made it home.

The Ford plant job was just a means to survive until Tomas could pursue his dream job in politics. He had a bachelor's degree in political science and thought someday he could be a campaign manager or even a candidate, but he couldn't get a foot in the door. He struggled to find any government work. The highest paying job with health insurance he *could* find was at the Ford assembly plant: $35,000 per year working the night shift. With student loans to pay, Tomas took the job and, to pay them back faster, roomed with his brother in Berwyn (a less expensive Chicago suburb).

But that commute. It was grueling. Tomas had to leave the house at 5 p.m. to arrive on time for his 7 p.m. shift. To make matters worse, the Ford plant was the size of 16 football fields. Workers with seniority could park closest to the assembly line entrance, while newcomer Tomas had the furthest possible parking spot. He described it as a "15-minute sprint to the entrance."

All the driving, sleep deprivation, and physically demanding work contributed to Tomas showing up late twice in his first two weeks on the job. On the second occasion, Tomas was fired.

"You can come here and get a union rep to sit in a hearing with you," the supervisor informed him dully, "But you will be terminated. They're not even going to pay you for the hour you're going to be here getting yelled at, so it's not worth even coming in [for a hearing]." Ford plant workers were unionized, but new employees needed to work a few months before earning union protections. At this point, he was still con-sidered a temp worker, easily fired.

With no income, no health insurance, and no job opportunities, Tomas figured he might as well return to his passion for politics. Back in Chicago, where legislative hopefuls and politicians running for city council need to collect 5,000 physical signatures to get their names on the ballot, he volunteered for campaigns and hoped his hard work would lead to a stable job.[5] Canvassing for signatures is time-consuming, demanding volunteer work. Tomas remembered he spent 40 to 50 hours a week canvassing in Chicago's blustery winter chill for three different candidates, and he was happy to get nearly 100 signatures a week. He performed so well that candidates started paying him $100 per day for his work.

The gambit paid off when Tomas was hired as chief of staff for an Illinois state legislator. This job, too, was a demanding one that required long hours with monthly trips to Springfield (the state capital), and at $30,000 a year without insurance; the pay was worse than Ford's but a lot better than volunteering. The heavy workload had Tomas constantly on his phone, responding to email, coordinating his boss' schedule, drafting press releases, and supervising volunteers; still, he was excited to be in politics and gaining job experience. Soon enough, if he excelled, he felt sure another opportunity would come along.

As Tomas joined the state congressional representative's staff in the spring and early summer of 2012, the Affordable Care Act (ACA) implementation was about to begin. Veteran public officials with significant campaign funding can afford to provide salary and benefits to their most crucial campaign staff, but those like Tomas's new boss just didn't have the funds to do so.[6] Worse, the whole job offer seemed like a bait-and-switch.

Incredulous, Tomas asked me, "Can you believe it's only been a month and my boss is cutting my pay?" He was supposed to be paid biweekly, but the legislator informed him a month into the job that paychecks were only going to come once a month. The amount on those checks would stay roughly the same. Tomas parsed this change: his annual income was actually going to be closer to $15,000 to $20,000 than the $30,000 he was promised.

After three months of receiving half his promised paycheck, Tomas started looking for work elsewhere. He liked the job but was tired of his economic precarity. With his experience at the Ford plant, volunteering for campaigns, and at the state legislature, Tomas had trouble finding other opportunities and became convinced he needed stronger educational credentials if he was going to make a career in politics. He decided to apply to law school. Tomas found the right program at a Chicago-area university with a four-year part-time program. After applying, taking the LSAT, and getting accepted, Tomas spent his final months before law school working at the legislator's office.

Although Medicaid expansion was underway at this point (fall 2013), Tomas was ambivalent about the ACA. Like many others in this book, his perceptions of the ACA were informed by his past experiences with the health care system. His were unpleasant, although not at first: as a child, he had insurance through his mother's employer, right up until she lost her job when Tomas was 18. It wasn't long before he had to put together his own health care safety net.

At age 20, Tomas felt a lump in his armpit. It was growing. He paid a couple hundred dollars to have a doctor examine it, only to learn that he should have the lump removed and tested for cancer. The doctor's office priced the biopsy at about $5,000 dollars—out of reach. With the help of family members in Mexico, Tomas found a doctor who would perform the biopsy for far less. He traveled by bus to Mexico, had the operation, and was relieved to learn that the tumor was benign. Slowly, Tomas paid back the $2,000 he borrowed from his brother for the procedure.

Tomas's beliefs about the health care safety net soured even more after visiting the Cook County emergency room with a high fever that was persistent for over 48 hours. Friends warned him to avoid County, but he went anyway and lived to regret it. "I was 24 or 25, and I was scared I was going to die," he explained of the decision. "I went to the emergency room, and they put my name down, took my vitals, and told me to wait. I ended up waiting 16 hours! I just got up and left." His fever lasted another day before ultimately subsiding.

The lesson Tomas learned was to avoid the county health care system altogether. Thereafter, he managed his health using home remedies or just forced himself to endure pain and discomfort. The final time he sought assistance from the health care safety net came when he experienced difficulty breathing and shortness of breath. Like Nick, in chapter 1, the inability to breathe pushed this ardent avoider to seek public assistance—this time, rather than going to Cook County's ER, Tomas visited a county health clinic in his neighborhood.

"They told me they needed to scan my lungs," he told me. "I didn't know any better so I got the test done and it turned out to be $1,500." Infuriated, he again found himself scrambling for cash to pay for what seemed like the most basic health care in the most austere settings. These experiences entrenched Tomas's desire to avoid the health care safety net.

Consequently, Tomas initially refused to apply for Medicaid. He'd gamble again, this time that he could remain healthy throughout law school.

* * *

The stakes changed when Tomas's father (Fernando) called, announcing, "I have Alzheimer's." Estranged from the rest of the family, Fernando asked, "Can I come stay with you?" Tomas reluctantly agreed. "He's kind of an asshole," he told me of his father.

In fact, Fernando was estranged from the family because he'd divorced Tomas's mother when, 27 years into their marriage, she was diagnosed with breast cancer. Fernando did not want to put forth the money or time to care for his wife, so he left her, returning to Mexico and remarrying. Tomas's new stepmother did not stay in the family long. After Fernando granted his bride access to his savings account, she withdrew all the money and ran off.

To recover from this financial loss, Fernando tried selling his home in Mexico. It was about then that he noticed his difficulty completing basic tasks. He would forget where he put things, lose his train of thought mid-conversation, and get lost on his way to and from the grocery store. A Mexican doctor confirmed: it was early-onset Alzheimer's, and Fernando's condition would only get worse over time. He was a US citizen, so he returned to Chicago to receive health care through Medicare.

The biggest challenge for Fernando at this point was finding a daily caretaker. Tomas's sisters had vowed never to speak to Fernando again, and they focused on caring for their mother.

"I was deciding what [law school] courses I was going to take in the fall when he called me," said Tomas. "I had no choice. No one was going to take him in. He's 76 years old. He cried and begged me on the phone to not put him in a retirement home. At the end of the day, he's still my dad." Despite the division and hardships his father had caused for the family, Tomas felt compelled to care for his father. With phrases like "I have no choice" and "he's still my dad," Tomas described a deeply inscribed sense of patriarchal obligation toward his father; the unsaid implication was that helping care for his cancer-stricken mother alongside his sisters was, by contrast, a choice rather than a requirement.

Here, we see the power of two interlocking social structures: family and the health care safety net. From this point forward, Tomas and his father's health care decisions would be inextricably linked, codependent. In fact, taking care of Fernando slowly took a toll on Tomas's health. It began with increasing social isolation. Tomas felt uncomfortable reaching out to friends for help, thinking it was an inappropriate favor to ask (although he pointed out that his father could go to the bathroom by himself and remain occupied by watching television). First, Fernando did not speak English. Second, Tomas feared his father might forget the identity of a drop-in caretaker and become scared or violent. Third, Tomas didn't have the time or money to properly compensate friends for their help.

After a few months of caring for his father, Tomas realized he was at a crossroads. As Alzheimer's can bring all sorts of health complications such as depression, malnutrition, dehydration, infections, and falls, Tomas knew it was only a matter of time before his father's conditions would deteriorate to the point where 24-hour caretaking was needed.[7] With law school on the horizon, he had to do something.

As the crisis worsened, Tomas turned to his social network. He started with his boss, asking whether if he knew of any state programs for elderly people with Alzheimer's. It was a good choice: his boss referred him to a state-funded nonprofit organization that provided no-cost day-care services for the elderly. Located in a northside Chicago neighborhood, it wasn't particularly convenient, but the nonprofit's bus service would transport elderly clients to and from their homes. Picking his father up at 7:30 a.m. and dropping him off at 5 p.m., the day care gave Tomas the flexibility to keep his part-time job as he started his part-time law school schedule. Those hours were more than enough time to fit in a few classes and possibly work from home in the evenings.

Unfortunately, it wasn't long before this arrangement fell apart. "I got a call from the day-care organization. They told me I had to pick up my dad," Tomas said over the phone.

"What? Why?" I asked.

"He was cursing at the staff, especially the women, and threatening them." This confirmed Tomas's instinct to avoid asking female friends, in particular, for help caring for his father. Alzheimer's hadn't stripped away Fernando's unapologetic sexism, with which he had so long spoken down to and derided the women in their family. It seemed to have intensified it.

Tomas had to leave work early to pick up Fernando, telling me, "I tried talking to him about what happened, but he could not recall any of the events." Staff at the day-care center warned Tomas that if his father didn't improve his behavior, they would not allow him to return. Sensing that it was only a matter of time before his father would be kicked out of the day care for good, Tomas was back to strategizing.

This time, finding alternative care for his father was much harder. Tomas had already exhausted all the help he could muster from his social network. His family was unwilling to get involved, and he did not want to burden his friends. The only alternative, Tomas concluded, was for him to find a less time-demanding job. His old boss referred him to a flexible-hours job at a Department of Motor Vehicles (DMV) office.

Two weeks later, Tomas made the job switch. The four-hour shift came with fewer responsibilities and a lighter workload than his political work, allowing Tomas to respond quickly to his father's needs. But it reactivated his social isolation. Now even work was devoid of regular meetings and casual workplace friendships. At the DMV, he was lucky if he occasionally got to interact with a customer. Mostly, his hours there were spent alone, in front of a computer. He had little time to do anything but work, study, and care for his father, so his social life dwindled.

When he started feeling depressed, Tomas searched online. He found an Alzheimer's support group that helped him feel less alone. And in it, he met Andrea, a working professional caring for her mother with Alzheimer's. They began dating, and Andrea helped Tomas smooth the gaps in his maddening schedule.

To the young man's delight, Fernando's behavior improved at the day-care center, and he was no longer in immediate danger of being kicked out. (Tomas still had his worries.) Thus, when law school was in session, Tomas became used to a new schedule that folded in assistance from the nonprofit and Andrea. He woke up at 6:30 a.m., because the day care's bus arrived any time between 6:40 a.m. and 8:45 a.m. Then he went to work at the DMV from 10 a.m. to 3 p.m., picked up his father, and dropped Fernando off at his girlfriend Andrea's house, where he'd stay as Tomas took his evening class at the law school. When classes ended at 9 p.m., he picked up his father and headed home.

Although the timing could be tight, Tomas had carved out a way to work, care for his father, date, and go to school. The only thing he couldn't accommodate was professional networking events. He simply did not have the time or energy to socialize.

"I was supposed to go out for drinks with some law school classmates on a Friday night," said Tomas. "It was 10 p.m. I just put my dad to sleep and went to charge my phone for a bit before I left the apartment. I sat on my couch as my phone charged and closed my eyes. When I opened them again it was 3 a.m.! I had all these text messages asking where I was, if I was all right. I was so embarrassed. My dad even came up to me and was like, 'Weren't you supposed to go out tonight?'"

Sleep-deprived again, as he had been in his time at Ford, Tomas was struggling physically. He had little time to shop for groceries or cook, so he mostly ate at drive-throughs. He would fall asleep when he tried to study and got dizzy at random hours of the day. Tomas gained weight and complained of stomachaches, likely the result of the stress and the food he ate.

To free up more time and improve his health, Tomas quit his job at the DMV to become an Uber driver. In theory, a ride-share driver can work as much or as little as they desire, so Tomas had complete control over his work schedule. The downsides stacked up, however: as independent contractors rather than employees, Uber drivers were ineligible for most worker benefits and protections, including a minimum wage, worker's compensation, and sick days,[8] and Tomas was required to pay for his own gas, car insurance, car payments, and vehicle maintenance. And the pay was unpredictable.

"There are good days and bad days," Tomas said of the job. "On good days, I'll earn $400 driving for four hours. On bad days, I'll earn $14. . . ." When requests for rides were low, Tomas had to drive more hours than anticipated. Once again, he found himself dozing off at the wheel, sometimes with customers in the back seat (like his health).

Things boiled over when Tomas started experiencing chest pains. His past attempts to ward off a health crisis had failed, and in his mind, desperate times called for desperate measures. With nowhere else to turn, Tomas decided to learn more about the ACA.

* * *

"Do you think that the Affordable Care Act will provide you adequate health care?" I asked Tomas as we drove along in his car.

"Sort of," Tomas replied. "It's weird to me, so I'd like to sit down with a social worker and let her break it down for me."

"You don't fear that signing up might harm you financially? Like with that bill you incurred all those years ago?"

"I'm a little worried, but I need to do more research and see what the bad things are and try to get around them. I'll figure it out." Tomas's deteriorating health changed his relationship with the health care safety net. Instead of avoiding it, Tomas was now strategizing, relying on lessons learned from past interactions to minimize the risks of seeking public assistance.

For instance, "With my dad, anytime the doctor tells me, 'He has to get this [procedure],' I ask, 'It's covered, right?'" If they respond with hesitation or say, "Yeah, it should be," Tomas continued, "I'm like 'Nah man, is it covered or not?'" Avoiding unexpected costs meant asking questions and insisting on getting answers from medical personnel.

A computer-savvy law student, Tomas found www.getcoveredillinois.gov through a Google search. The official website for information about the ACA in Illinois, it listed a calendar of Chicago-area outreach events where he could ask questions of a health navigator face-to-face. There was a health fair coming up at high school gymnasium in his neighborhood, with walk-in enrollment appointments available for a few hours on a Saturday morning. I tagged along, stamping next to Tomas in my heavy coat, hat, and gloves on this chilly early spring day.

"Good morning, how are you?" asked a health navigator near the door.

"Good morning," said Tomas, staring at the piles of paperwork on her desk.

"Do you have any questions?" she prompted.

"Well, I never really had health insurance on my own," Tomas explained, "so I'm not really sure what to ask."

"That's OK," the navigator assured him, "there's different options. There's the marketplace with four different plans: bronze, silver, gold, and platinum. Depending on which one you choose, the coverage will be 60/40, 70/30, 90/10." Already, she had assumed too much, referring to coinsurance and the insurance–beneficiary cost split on medical bills. Tomas was unfamiliar with this terminology and glanced at me with confusion as the navigator continued. "There is also Medicaid that has been extended for adults. So, if you don't have insurance, depending on your income, you might be able to qualify for assistance."

"Well, I've been driving for Uber but haven't been making that much money."

"Then you might be eligible. We'll have to crunch the numbers. Another option is that if you are under the age of 26 you could still get covered through your parents' insurance."

"Neither of my parents have health insurance," Tomas replied.

"OK, then Medicaid may be your best option. There's also catastrophic plans, where you pay a low premium. But let's see what your income is, then go from there."

The health navigator pulled out her laptop and then looked up glumly. "I'm sorry that the internet isn't working, so I can't do this application with you. Could you write down your contact information so I can follow up with you?" she asked.

A few days later, the navigator did call. She booked him an appointment at her office in a nonprofit health clinic. Again, I accompanied Tomas.

"Do you have an ID on you?" asked the receptionist when we checked in.

"I do," said Tomas.

"Are you a citizen?"

"Yes."

"Are you employed?"

"Kind of."

"That's OK," said the receptionist. He surely wasn't the first.

The navigator who greeted us after a few minutes in the waiting room was not the same woman from the health fair. "Hi, I'm Sarah," the navigator began before explaining, "Beatrice, who called you, had to step out today so I'm here to help you in her place. She said you were interested in health care?"

In her office, Sarah asked, "Now, you wanted to do the health care, or you wanted to do the Medicaid?" When Tomas answered, "I'm not really sure which one," she described the former and noted, "You'll be limited to our facilities in Cook County," and then, "But if I sign you up for Medicaid though, you can use it anywhere."

"Oh, OK, so then let's do Medicaid I guess," said Tomas.

"You'll do the Medicaid?" the navigator asked.

"Yes," Tomas answered, and they got started creating an online account for him on the Medicaid application website. A window popped up, and the navigator told him, "Now, before you complete the application, you must read the following penalty affidavit and provide certification of understanding and acceptance." He agreed, and she read out the official, vaguely threatening bureaucratic text: "Do you understand that any information on this form is subject to verification by federal, state, and local officials? If you give false or misleading information, you are subject to criminal or civil prosecutions?"

"Yes," Tomas replied.

"Do you also understand that if you are prosecuted for fraud you will be required to repay any amount wrongfully received, and be disqualified from the program?"

"Yes," Tomas replied again.

"Are you applying for food stamps, cash assistance, or just medical?" she asked.

"Just medical."

They moved on to questions about income, citizenship, and household characteristics. When Tomas entered information about employment, Sarah paused. "I thought you said you didn't have a job."

"I drive for Uber sometimes. It's not a steady job, and it's not a lot of money."

The crucial moment came when it was time for Tomas to enter a figure for his monthly income. The navigator said he could just "give a ball-park estimate," but hearing that he was paid weekly and his income fluctuated, she suggested he tally up his most recent weeks' checks. The Uber app gave him the numbers, so he entered $1,432.48.

They completed the online application, the navigator made photocopies of Tomas's ID and Social Security card, and we left. "You should hear from the Medicaid office in a few weeks," the navigator said on our way out.

One month later, Tomas was rejected by Medicaid. The threshold for an individual adult's monthly income as $1,366, and a few "good" weeks with Uber had put him $66.48 over. Tomas was livid. The month before, his income was $863! Bad timing, bad luck, or bad information—if the navigator had known the monthly cutoff, they might have averaged his income or just waited to apply in leaner weeks—no matter, this is the kind of close call that comes with means-tested government programs. Some people, just dollars above destitute, will be rejected.

With his health crisis still unresolved, Tomas went to healthcare.gov (the website printed on his Medicaid rejection letter). Maybe he could afford one of the subsidized private health insurance plans. He could not. The cheapest plan option, after government subsidies, was $110 a month.

"It turns out the Affordable Care Act ain't so affordable," Tomas complained from back on square one. As before, Tomas responded to this disappointment by working harder, longer hours and saving money just in case. He cut his study hours and networking at law school to drive more hours for Uber. It took six months to save up for a medical consultation about his chest pains and dizziness, only to have to cancel two appointments in a row because of emergencies with his father.

"I guess if I keel over and end up in the ER, I know I have money to at least cover some of the bill." Tomas laughed.

* * *

Tomas's rejected Medicaid application had short- and long-term consequences. More hours driving ride-share left fewer hours for studying and networking. His grades suffered, while his work and commitments to caring for his father robbed him of time to join other law students in trying to line up the prestigious summer positions with law firms, corporations, or government agencies that build professional connections and sometimes turn into full-time job offers upon graduation. His health continued to deteriorate as he gained weight, risking longer-term health problems, but there was little he could do about it. All his resources seemed to have been gobbled up by the end of each day.

The interlocking structures of gendered family obligations, economic precarity, and the means-tested Medicaid income eligibility cutoff contributed to Tomas being uninsured for the full three-year duration of this study. Tomas rationalized it as bad luck. From a sociological perspective, however, his circumstances stemmed from an interlocking set of social structures that iteratively blocked Tomas's access to health insurance from one situation to the next.

"I Don't Think He Understands the Financial Risk of Being Uninsured"

Renee was a 22-year-old fourth-year college student who wanted to make a difference in the world.

"I want to open doors for people to get into academia and higher education," she declared when we met in 2013. Renee had an older sister who finished college and was attending graduate school. Her parents were working-class Mexican immigrants. Initially, Renee found college overwhelming, but she blossomed through her involvement with Latino student organizations. Her attachment to these student groups helped her muster up the courage to speak up in class when more privileged students spoke derisively about immigrants or Mexicans. At one point, Renee turned down a $5,000 scholarship from a corporation whose CEO advocated for increased border patrol. Renee was growing into a spirited and socially conscious campus leader.

Her activism started at home where, despite her parents' objections, Renee took additional student loans to pay for housing off campus. The decision was strategic—a declaration of independence. She said her parents expressed little support for her educational aspirations and expected her to remain at home to serve them until she married. "They've always tried controlling everything I do," Renee complained. "And when I tell them I'm not young anymore, that I have a job, an apartment, they say 'That's not how we raised you! You're so ungrateful!'"

"How would that make you feel?" I asked.

"Bad, but I disagreed. It still feels bad, though, to hear your parents talk like that."

Despite many arguments, Renee was trying to follow in the footsteps of her older sister (Sylvia), who was enrolled in a PhD program at a research university on the West Coast. Sylvia explained: "With my parents, I've learned to just do what I want; there's no reasoning with them.

"I don't argue with my parents because it's a waste of time," said Renee. "I'd rather spend my time on something else."

Renee's independence from her family also meant she was uninsured. Her experiences in the past made her wary of seeking information about the ACA when it debuted in the fall of 2013. She cited a trip to a medical office for low-income clients.

"When you go into county clinics," Renee claimed, "they don't tell you how much things cost, or they tell you it costs a certain amount but when you're done it ends up being more expensive." Once, when she was living with her parents, she had gone in for a $90 physical, but when a nurse insisted that she needed an asthma test ("You need it," she remembered the nurse urging. "You want to be able to breathe, right?"), the bill was $300. At the time, her father was out of work with a back injury, and the bill was a genuine financial crisis for their family.

When it came to the ACA, Renee's memory left her skeptical and disinterested. She told me she was "just planning to take care of myself, avoid getting sick, and find a job that provides health insurance." She couldn't afford another safety net that landed her in deeper financial trouble.

* * *

A year later, in the fall of 2014, Renee was still uninsured but living in radically different circumstances. She delayed graduation by a semester to finish a required course, but her campus job expired at the end of the academic calendar year. She was unemployed but didn't yet have her degree, and employers weren't biting. She begrudgingly moved back in with her parents.

Sylvia suggested Renee consider applying for Medicaid, although that idea was vetoed by their father.

"My dad files me as a dependent on his tax returns, and he's afraid that if I get Obamacare it will lower his tax benefits. He doesn't want me to enroll," Renee lamented.

"Does your dad know the financial risk of you getting sick?" I asked.

"He does. Even the guy from H&R Block who does his taxes told him to let me sign up, because they would have to pay a penalty of a couple hundred dollars for me being uninsured. But my dad said no. In his eyes, it's better to pay a couple hundred dollars once a year instead of every month."

Renee's father, a mechanic, paid $500 a month to get health insurance for himself and his wife through his employer. Adding Renee to his plan would be an additional $300 a month, too costly for a family with a monthly income of $2,800 and a mortgage to pay.

Despite numerous attempts to explain that she qualified for Medicaid, which would come at no cost to him, Renee's father refused to listen.

"Have you considered just applying on your own?" I asked, but she didn't have the privacy to go against her parents' wishes when she needed them for her basic needs—food and shelter. She worried, "If I get something in the mail about Obamacare, they'll know I signed up." She was in no situation to risk being cut off from her parents' support, and she felt lonesome because her mother always backed up her father's patriarchal expectations.

"My mom wants to talk to me and vent about him when I don't want to listen to her vent. [Then] she gets mad at me and tells me I'm ungrateful." Renee's parental pressures included both her father's patriarchal pressures to obey him and her mother's gendered pressure to meet her emotional needs.

When I spoke to Renee's sister Sylvia, I asked: "How do you make sense of your father?"

"I don't," she said quickly. "It just doesn't make sense to me. I think he doesn't help Renee because of the added cost, but I don't think he understands the financial risk of being uninsured. He thinks we're all healthy because there hasn't been a need to go to the hospital." Sylvia also recognized that gendered dynamics were a problem for the sisters: "My dad also doesn't know about the reproductive health issues that we go through, and his ignorance allows him to say we don't need it." The patriarchal expectations of their household prevented Renee from having her health needs recognized and met, even though it would cost nothing. And her economic dependence on her parents prevented her from any alternative.[9] She remained uninsured.

The male-dominated home also damaged Renee's mental health. Her father verbally abused her through criticism and unsolicited sexist advice. "It's stressful just being around them," said Renee of her parents, "and it's harder with my sister away. [Our father] always asks when we're going to get married, when we're going to have kids. Sylvia doesn't come home because of that." No longer willing to accept or even entertain their parents' unsolicited "advice," Sylvia stayed at hotels or rented sublet apartments over holiday breaks.

"When I disagree, they guilt-trip us," Renee revealed in another moment, "saying that they've sacrificed so much for us and that we're ungrateful."

"What does your mom think about your dad's behavior?" I asked, although she'd already indicated her mother frequently wanted to "vent" about her father.

"She doesn't like it either," answered Renee. "He gives her attitude and gets mad at her for the smallest things. For example, my mom was doing internet research on trade schools and community college. She wanted to go back to school and get a job, but he shut her down saying she was too old and too dumb."

The few conversations Renee had with her father only produced more pain and frustration. "My dad opens up to me about being tired about work, the neighborhood, how it's changing, when his coworkers get fired or laid off," Sylvia said. "I try to use these opportunities to tell him he should help my mom and stop being so hard on her. He responds saying, 'Well, I had a long day at work, plus all *you* do is sit down and read.' What am I supposed to say to that?"

At one point, older sister Sylvia had tried opening up to their parents about her mental health struggles in graduate school. A first-generation student at a prestigious university, Sylvia struggled with social adjustment. "When I shared my struggles with depression and anxiety, they said, 'No, you don't have that.' They don't understand the importance of mental health care. They think it's a waste of money and that doctors just want to take your money." Sylvia's father thought the same of graduate school, going out of his way to call it a waste of time. "He literally asked me, 'If you go to graduate school, who is going to cook and do the dishes in your home when you get married?' It's hard for him to grasp that women can have careers," Sylvia concluded with a blank stare.

The sexism, emotional blackmail, and patriarchal dynamics brought together the social structures of the family, inadequate health care, and sexism in a way that powerfully constrained Renee's access to health insurance. When Renee resisted, verbal abuse and sexism disciplined her into abiding by the family's patriarchal hierarchy—for a time, at least. She was still strategizing, trying to figure out how to convince her dad to change his mind. "I'm going to try and approach him on one of his days off, when he's gardening or doing a chore," Renee told me of her plan. "It's easiest to talk with him when he is occupied with something else."[10]

With one course to go before she could graduate, Renee's career and future plans were on hold. "I'm not applying to graduate school right now, but I'm thinking of going into public policy or nonprofit management. I'm just focusing on finishing school, getting a job right now, and talking to my dad about getting health insurance."

* * *

When I followed up with Renee in 2016, she was still living with her parents, unemployed, and uninsured. She and her dad never had that conversation about Medicaid.

"Why didn't you talk to your dad?" I asked.

"I knew it was going to be an argument, and I don't like arguing because it affects my mental health. I just write poetry about it to destress." I was puzzled by the contrast in Renee's demeanor with the spirited and civic-minded version young woman I met in 2013.

"Why poetry?"

"Six months ago, I was raped."

We both fell silent. After a few moments, I said, "Oh my god, I'm so sorry to hear that. That's terrible."

"It's OK. Writing poetry gets me through anxiety attacks. It happened at a friend's house. He was a friend from one of the student organizations I was part of at school. He had roommates, but when I came over to watch a movie, no one was there. He threw himself on me. I didn't press charges. It took a long time for me to process everything, and by that time it was too late. I still haven't graduated. I still haven't found work. Friends and people at school kept asking about me, but I didn't want to repeat telling the story over and over again. It weighs a lot on me."

Like Tomas, Renee's sacrifices for her family patriarch had impeded her ability to care for her own help. Renee understood herself and her problems as insignificant and undeserving of help, and so she did not reach out for help from friends, family, police, or medical personnel after her sexual assault. She didn't want to be a burden on others, so she carried the burden of her trauma with her every moment of every day.

A month after her assault, Renee was walking home with a friend one night when they witnessed a woman being assaulted in a parking lot. "We called the police, but they didn't come." Witnessing the assault retriggered her own trauma. The anxiety crippled her ability to concentrate or perform basic tasks. She rarely left her room.

To find solace, Renee visited an old high school friend who lived in a nearby college town. They went to a party, but "I wasn't feeling well, so I went back to the apartment," said Renee. Her friend stayed behind, and when Renee woke up, her host was nowhere to be found. She called frantically, but no one answered. It was late morning before Renee's friend finally came home and told her she had passed out, waking up with a friend on top of her. Police officers came to the apartment, interviewed both Renee and her friend, and took a report on the assault. Renee, who just could not escape the shadow of sexual violence, continued to experience panic attacks.

Shockingly and shamefully, Renee's repeated experiences of sexual assault—both her own and others'—were not unique. Every 98 seconds, a person in the United States experiences sexual assault, and only six out of every 1,000 perpetrators will end up in prison for the assault.[11]

When Renee finally told her sister everything, Sylvia acknowledged that their parents had dismissed her mental health problems. Renee wasn't "crazy" to think her parents might blame her for being raped. Nonetheless, she urged Renee to tell them: she really needed health insurance and mental health services. Renee refused.

"My parents are still helping me with money for food and things," Renee told me. "I'm just praying that I can get a job that provides me health insurance."

Renee's social isolation and trauma exacerbated the difficulty of finishing school and finding a job. Her inability to process or explain her year of unemployment to friends or potential employers made it particularly tough to get hired or leverage social networks into an interview.[12] For the time being, Renee relied heavily on help from Sylvia.

Sylvia eventually found a sliding-scale mental health provider and helped Renee pay the $300 to get an appointment and fill an antianxiety prescription. Without regular mental health access (even the access afforded back when she was a full-time student), the medications were the only type of formal help Renee received.

The sexual assault amplified all the intersections that already disempowered Renee and impeded her from getting help. Inadequate health care, gender, and family support socially isolated Renee, trapping her in a home where she was expected to continue abiding by her parents' patriarchal expectations and ignoring her own needs.

When our interview ended, we left the coffee shop and walked out onto the street. I asked Renee what she had planned for the rest of the day. "I'm taking my dog to get a free flu shot." As we parted, she joked ruefully, "It's a shame that my dog can get health care but I can't."

*   *   *

In 2017, Renee had gotten a job (albeit temporary and without health insurance benefits). Her sister helped her find a program that provided 10 free sessions with a licensed mental health counselor. Renee used up her free visits quickly, but the sessions helped her find productive ways to cope and manage her anxiety.

"I'm still in the process of forgiving," said Renee in reference to the man who assaulted her, "but it's been hard, because it's painful to talk about."

She was taking steps toward regaining a sense of control over her life. She finally took the last class she needed to graduate, and she was constantly applying for jobs. Hobbies like art and yoga helped her manage stress and anxiety. Although she lived at home, her parents, as is common among female sexual violence survivors of Mexican heritage, knew nothing about her sexual assault.[13] In fact, she told me, she didn't speak to her parents very much anymore. She was trying everything possible to achieve economic independence, but until then, she survived through a steady routine of part-time work and spending time in her room with her pet, applying for jobs, and losing herself in her hobbies. Renee told me that getting a job with health insurance benefits was going to help her turn a corner.

Cutting the Umbilical Cord

Originally from Janesville, Wisconsin, 23-year-old culinary worker Tina Bailey had lived in Chicago for five years when we met at a social event in Little Village. She was a young white woman in a predominantly male industry, and she had just one year in culinary school under her belt. Her bakery job paid just above minimum wage. "It's tough," Tina said in that first conversation, "but my mom helps me a lot by paying bills here and there. I'm also on her health insurance, so that helps."

Tina's parents divorced when she was a toddler, and she had never been close with her father. Her brother worked as a cook in their hometown, and their mother, a licensed therapist, begrudgingly supported their career aspirations (although she would have preferred they had attended college instead).

When the ACA rolled out in the fall of 2013, Tina saw no reason to learn about it: she was insured through her mother. Circumstances changed six months later when Tina's mom suddenly dropped her from her health insurance plan.

"She took it off because it was cheaper for her," Tina explained. "She took my brother off, too. She's not under financial stress; she owns a home and a new car; it's more like this is her way of telling us to do our own thing. She's been pushing me and my brother to become more independent, and I guess this is her way of cutting the umbilical cord. She warned us she was going to do this."

"Did you try to convince her to change her mind?" I asked.

"We had a very adult conversation. She simply said she was going to take me off because it was cheaper and that I should get health insurance for myself. That was pretty much it."

"How do you feel about that?"

"It's scary. I'm not sure what I'm going to do now. She's really trying to push us out of the nest. To be honest, that was the last thing that was tying me to her."

By withdrawing support, Tina's mother sought to motivate her daughter into acquiring health insurance, as if a lack of motivation were the sole reason Tina was uninsured. What it actually did was leave Tina more vulnerable to a major economic crisis. When that crisis arrived two months later, when Tina lost her job, she turned for help instead from her boyfriend's family.

* * *

Unemployed and uninsured, Tina at least had the support of her boyfriend, Drew. They had only been dating for six months, but 26-year-old Drew (Latino) helped as much as he could. It wasn't much, given he still lived with his mother and earned too little at his job selling cell phones to be fully independent, but Drew convinced his mother to offer Tina room in their home.

After moving in, Tina learned that Drew's mother (Ruth) ran a childcare center out of the home she owned. Before his untimely death, her husband was a well-paid carpenter. Now, Drew's income and what Ruth made through the in-home childcare business provided just enough to pay the mortgage and other living expenses. Drew and Ruth lived paycheck to paycheck.

The day-care business was aboveboard, having met all the state of Illinois guidelines, from background checks to square footage, a clean home inspection report, and a review of the neighborhood's service population.[14] As a lone operator, Ruth was licensed to care for a maximum of 12 children in her facility on the first floor of their home.[15] When Tina moved in, Ruth saw it as a temporary opportunity to generate more income and asked if Tina might help out with the childcare center. "She would pay me in cash $180 per week," Tina remembered, and she figured, "It was better than nothing." With a second staff member, the childcare center could take care of more kids, and Tina was happy that Ruth only expected her to help with cooking their meals.

Ruth also urged Tina to apply for food stamps and Medicaid, giving her the information she needed to go apply at the public aid office. Tina had no previous experience with the social safety net or the county health care system, and she didn't know what to expect. "I had to physically go to this public aid office, and the line was out of this world. If you get there early, you're still late. I waited four hours. It was ridiculous."

"How did things go?" I asked.

"I went into the meeting with the caseworker, and she was like, 'You just need to have a signed or written letter saying how much you earn.' Ruth gave me a signed letter, and I got food stamps."

"What about your Medicaid application?"

"That took a long time to process. I was able to get on food stamps quickly, but a month and a half later, I learned they rejected my Medicaid."

"Did they explain why?"

"They said I needed an actual payroll check to prove that I was earning my money. I was able to use the rest of the food stamps I got, but when I went to renew my food stamps, they now rejected my food stamps application, too. The problem was they knew I was working at the childcare center, because Ruth has my name listed as someone helping her. They know I have income from there, and since I don't have check stubs, I have no way of proving how much I'm earning."

The "tough love" decision Tina's mom made to drop her children from her health insurance set off a chain of events that even Tina's motivation couldn't overcome. She had risen to the occasion, finding a place to live, an informal job, and people to help her apply for assistance getting health care and food subsidies. Rather than become more financially independent, though, Tina ended up more dependent on a different family. The combination of family structural dynamics with an unstable and precarious culinary labor market severely constrained Tina's ability to get on her feet.

* * *

In 2015, things changed again. Drew got a city government job that boosted his income to $80,000. Drew and Tina were able to rent a modest apartment by themselves in Little Village and help support Ruth with some of her bills. Shortly after the couple's move, Tina found a job teaching cooking classes in an affluent neighborhood for $22,000 a year, no health insurance benefits.

Her new income put Tina just above Medicaid's income eligibility cutoff, but she received an email from healthcare.gov and explored options through the ACA. Unfortunately, the email turned out to be a phishing scam. As soon as she entered her personal information, the computer screen was flooded with advertisements. The experience left Tina afraid and confused over which online websites were legitimate sources. At the same time, resuming work in a kitchen compelled Tina to prepare for an on-the-job injury: "you have to worry about cuts or burns. I work with knives all the time and have experience, so I'm not worried about myself. My biggest fear is the people walking around me with knives or boiling pots. I trust myself, but I don't trust other people. It just takes one second for that knife to go somewhere else, and that terrifies me because if I have to go into an ambulance, that's $1,000."

"Sounds very stressful," I said.

"Yeah, I think about it a lot, and my mom she's been telling me I need to get health insurance or I'll be fined, which is bullshit. If people like me don't have health insurance, it's because we can't afford it."

Tina's mother again adopted her "natural growth" parenting style by issuing a directive to acquire health insurance or risk paying a fine (which, at the time in Illinois, was $90, waived for those living below the poverty line).[16] Despite this, and despite the fact that Tina underscored the importance of having health insurance as she worked in a physically demanding and dangerous environment, Tina's mother made no further effort to help her find health insurance.

"Does the threat of the fine make you want to learn more about the ACA?" I asked Tina.

"Yes and no. I've been without health insurance for nine months, and nothing's happened. But it also concerns me because I really need to be able to see a doctor if something bad happens."

"Has your experience with food stamps and Medicaid changed your perspective on government?" I asked.

"Again, yes and no, because when I got food stamps that one time, it helped, but then I got denied. It's just confusing."

Tina had begun using a small health clinic Ruth suggested, where uninsured patients could get sliding-scale care. "It got me a prescription for birth control," Tina said, "I only paid $30. . . . It's just a clinic. They can't do major surgeries or operations, but it's there." Tina's new kinship network (Drew's mom) inadvertently blocked her from enrolling in Medicaid, yet it also conveyed information on where to find cheaper out-of-pocket sources of care.

Toward the end of our conversation, Tina asked if I had any information on which website was the right place to find information about the ACA. After being phished, she was mistrustful. I obliged, showing her the heathcare.gov site on my laptop. "Interesting," she commented. She needed to get to work, so we couldn't explore the website further, but I asked whether she would allow me to sit down with her as she explored the website. She agreed and we met up a week later at a downtown library.

Tina started by following all the prompts on the website. She began by entering her zip code, her county, the names of everyone in her household, her age, gender, whether she was pregnant. "It's asking how much my income will be," Tina said staring at the screen and thinking it over. "Well, I earn $1,800 a month, which comes out to $21,600 a year."

While we waited for the site to generate Tina's eligible insurance plans, a window popped up alerting "You may be eligible for a tax credit." The plans loaded, and Tina scrolled to find the one with the lowest monthly premium. A Blue Choice Bronze PPO plan with a $129 per month premium and $6,000 deductible was the cheapest option we could find.[17]

"That's too much," Tina said.

She didn't understand what a deductible was, so she typed it into Google and read aloud: "A specified amount of money the insured must pay before an insurance company will file a claim. What!?" she exclaimed, shaking her head. "I *definitely* can't afford that." Her exploration of the healthcare.gov website ended in 15 minutes with a firm decision to remain uninsured.

* * *

Tina, in fact, was uninsured for the full three years of this study. In our last conversation, in 2016, she cited the cost as her reason for remaining uninsured.

"One hundred twenty-nine dollars is so expensive, and the deductible is way too high," she said, "I don't even see the doctor that much, and I don't want to pay for something that I'm not really going to use."

"Have you paid any penalty for it?"

"I ended up paying $600 when I filed my taxes, but that's still cheaper than $129 per month."

We were talking on the phone, and I could hear Tina's congestion. She had the flu, and it was bad.

"What are you doing to get better?" I asked.

"I'm just trying to let it naturally go away. I'm terrified of going to the doctor. If I can avoid it, I do. But if I ever get to the point where I can't continue, then I'll go. What's most terrifying to me is the waiting. Just sitting there waiting and not knowing what's wrong with you. I'm still going to the sliding-scale place, but if I have something serious, I know they won't be able to help me."

In these few sentences, Tina illuminates why so many uninsured tend to seek help from the health care safety net only during a major health crisis. When people live in fear of going to the doctor due to concerns over financial cost or harrowingly long waits, they only seek public assistance in an absolute worst-case scenario. Such outcomes burden not only the uninsured but also the health care organizations providing them crisis care rather than preventive and chronic care. In addition, Tina was constrained by the interlocking structures of the labor market (especially the low wages and precarity of the culinary industry), family (her mother's tough-love approach and Ruth's mistake in not issuing pay stubs), and health care that had proved overly expensive and even included an identity scam. At a time when she should have been eligible to receive significant support, Tina continued to face difficulties getting health coverage under the ACA.

Fortunately, Tina did not experience a major health crisis during the three years of this study, but her circumstances at the time of our last conversation left her in a vulnerable position. Her job was dangerous, plagued by back and knee problems, as well as cuts and burns. She depended on her partner to share the burden of their housing, food, and utility expenses, raising the stakes of a breakup (and leading her to go along with his mother's wishes, which had made her ineligible for Medicaid in the first place).

Tina's experience also illuminated the workings of race and class, which contributed to the different kinds of family obligations she encountered over the three years. Tina's relationship with her mother represented a white middle-class form of family obligation, in which Tina failed to meet expectations and was penalized with estrangement and the withdrawal of support. Her mother's plan to make Tina more independent actually transferred Tina's sense of family obligation to her Latino boyfriend and his mother—this transference of racialized, classed, and gendered family obligations only further restricted Tina's chances at insurance and financial independence.

Winston Harrison

Winston was a 32-year-old white male born and raised in a rural part of New York state, and his case exemplifies the drastically different family obligations of uninsured white men.

When we met, it was 2013. Winston lived with his girlfriend in the gentrifying Logan Square neighborhood and worked at a printmaking shop. It was a small niche business that paid $9 an hour with no insurance and involved hard physical work, hand-binding books or kneeling to operate an old-fashioned printing press.

Winston had been uninsured for seven years, and he seemed OK with it. His mother was a different story: "The conversation's always been, 'Well what if this happens? . . . What if *this* happens?'" he said, imitating her concern. "But health insurance has always been so expensive." Winston's mother suggested he get at least a catastrophic plan (with a $10,000 deductible), but he refused, confident he could find alternative forms of care to meet his needs. Unlike Tina's mother, Winston's did pressure him to pursue a safer or better-paid career or take better care of himself. Winston was too old to be covered under his mother's family health insurance plan, so she kept at it, trying to persuade rather than compel him to acquire health insurance.

He did seem to do all he could to avoid paying for expensive medical care, and he sought physical care in nontraditional settings. For example, when he could save up enough funds, he visited acupuncturists to treat the back and shoulder pain that came with his job. But he'd been fortunate, and unlike other respondents, he'd never had any memorable experiences with the health care safety net. In fact, Winston had never even visited an emergency room. To this point, he had lived a relatively crisis-free life.

To his credit, Winston recognized this was an unusual string of good luck and class privilege: "You know, health insurance is something I've never really had to think about. So, when I think about past experiences, I think they were good. We had a family doctor that I always saw where

I grew up until I was 18. The same doctors and same dentist my entire time there. Everything was good. It was never a discussion until now."

In the event of a serious medical emergency, friends had taught him he could go to the Logan Square health clinic (he never had). His sole experience interacting with a health care facility in Chicago was when he went to get free sexually transmitted infection testing at a Cook County health clinic near downtown. "A friend recommended it to me," he began. "The guy took me in the office and showed me all these gory pictures of STDs [sexually transmitted diseases]. I thought that was totally unnecessary. It was like they were trying to scare me into not having sex. I also had to wait two weeks for an AIDS test result, which was negative, but scary to wait for." Not a trauma like those shared in other interviews, this experience was recounted as an inconvenience.

I brought up the ACA, and Winston expressed some skepticism but conceded he wasn't avidly following the news or trying to learn about it. Mostly, he distrusted the health system's profit motives: "I'm a bit skeptical of the health insurance companies," Winston said, "they're in the position to make the most money from all of this. My sense is they are going to try and get as much money from you while providing as little as they can. That's just the nature of business." Seeing little need for health insurance and wanting to make his meager paychecks stretch, Winston intended to remain uninsured for the foreseeable future.

* * *

When I reconnected with Winston a year and a half later, in 2015, he was a new father, was engaged to his girlfriend, and was living in a rural town in Massachusetts.[18] His fiancée (also white) found a lucrative job there—a six-figure professional salary—and so Winston was willing to prioritize her career. Getting married meant upward mobility for Winston, even though he was now uninsured and unemployed. His only health insurance option was to seek subsidized private insurance through the Massachusetts state exchange, but remaining uninsured was not burdensome on his family, nor did it stem from his need to shoulder family burdens. His concerns and needs continued to be met and addressed, no matter what.

"My son was born in Chicago, and the cheapest option was for my son and I was to go on a plan together, rather than put the whole family on my wife's plan at work." After moving to Massachusetts, his wife's new job provided low-cost health insurance for her and their son, but not Winston. He was in no hurry to apply for Medicaid or seek out an ACA plan, but unlike the last time we spoke, he had a new rationale for this reluctance—easily traceable, as we spoke further, to the political leanings of his new wife's family, who now lived nearby.

"My fear [about enrolling] is that I would be paying into a system and not really getting much out of it," Winston said in words I heard from other respondents, including my focal group, Latinos. "Like, when I was insured in Chicago for a few months, the deductible was high, I never used it, but had to pay, and even if I did use it, I would have been forced to pay for most of my doctor's visits anyway. The deductible was $6,000, which meant I had to pay that amount before any coverage kicked in."

Winston now spoke of the ACA as an unfair tax asking healthy people to pay for less healthy and more disadvantaged populations to get care. "The ACA is relying on healthy people like me to pay into the system," Winston charged. "I understand people need health care and can't get it, but the government has no business doing that on the backs of healthy people."[19] I learned quickly that two aspects of Winston's move to rural Massachusetts triggered this new line of thinking: it was not only his wife's extended family and their heavy involvement in politics but also his experiences with the health care safety net in Massachusetts.

It all began when Winston started seeking help for his debilitating back pain. On some days, the pain was so severe it rendered him immobile. "My old job," at the print shop, "required a lot of circular shoulder motions and cranking heavy machinery, and your posture is not the best." Winston consulted a doctor in his town to diagnose the pain as it spread from his lower back to his right leg. "They thought it was sciatic pain. [But] my whole right leg would just be out of commission. It hasn't gone away, and having a toddler running around was difficult to deal with."

After days of internet searches and phone calls, Winston was unable to find a health insurance plan that would provide much coverage for the physical therapy recommended to treat his pain. "Money is the bottom line here," Winston said. "Health care is expensive for people like *me* so that *other* people can get health care."

"What makes you think that?" I asked.

"It's just, when you go by health clinics or county hospitals, and just see who is using that health care, it's sick people who don't have money," he explained, "and a lot of them are not paying it."

"How do you know they can't pay for it?" I asked.

"My wife and I make about $100,000 a year now, and even we can't pay for it. Where do you think they're getting the money for it? It has to come from somewhere. It comes on the backs of people like us."

Winston casually used "us" and "them" terms, deploying his implicitly racialized identification with a segment of the population that he characterizes as unfairly burdened with the needs of the poor and the sick. Research on stereotypes and the welfare state has repeatedly demonstrated how deservingness is often synonymous with whiteness when we talk about public aid in the United States.[20] In contrast to Tomas, whose family made him feel obligated to sacrifice his own health and career prospects to care for his father, Winston's status as a white male in a white family with class resources produced a different set of family obligations. That is, Winston now felt an obligation to contest a health care system perceived as unfair by white people with more resources— like his in-laws and, by extension, him.

"When I interviewed you a year and a half ago, you didn't use this language of 'paying into a system for sick people and getting nothing out of it,'" I pointed out. "What has changed that made you start using that language?"

Winston paused, taking a few seconds before answering.

"I started being around my wife's extended family," Winston concluded, "who are involved in local government. My aunt ran for mayor of the town and lost, but I would go out to her events and talk to people, and it was there that I talked to people who helped me understand what was going on with the ACA."

The civic life in Winston's new politically conservative rural town provided him with a new interpretive frame for making sense of the ACA and a man's obligations to family. "It's such a backwards system," he said of the program known as Obamacare. "I feel like we're being penalized for having more income. Even if I signed up for one of their plans, the system would still treat me like I'm uninsured." The only difference Winston could see in being uninsured or getting an ACA plan was that one would force him to pay for others to access health care. He remained uninsured, even as his own health crisis escalated.

* * *

Winston tried using friend and family networks to find a secure job that provided health insurance benefits, but nothing materialized. Thus, when we talked for the final time in 2016, I learned that his solution to his increasingly painful back and leg problems was to give up his job search, become a stay-at-home father, and learn techniques to manage his pain. His family was just fine with this arrangement.

"I just stay at home with the kids," he said. "Thankfully my wife earns enough and can work from home on most days." Winston developed a pain management lifestyle that included acupuncture appointments, stretching, yoga, and meditation.[21] On the most painful days, Winston could get a steroid shot to numb the pain—his wife paid the bill.

As it did for the others in this chapter, race, class, and gender materialized through family obligations to shape Winston's health insurance access. Initially, his mother pressured him to acquire health insurance but stopped short of penalizing him when he did not. When Winston became closer to his wife's family in Massachusetts, he was socialized into a local political culture that taught him the language and ideology for opposing the ACA on ideological grounds. With this more politicized, racialized, and class-inflected sense of family obligations, Winston now felt a powerful family obligation to abstain from the ACA and, through his wife, do so while still managing his extreme pain.

This case also illuminates the importance of place, as Chicago is a predominantly liberal Democratic city whereas Winston's rural Massachusetts town was predominantly conservative Republican.[22] Civic life and ACA outreach in these places differed considerably, and this definitely matters when trying to understand uninsured people's orientations to the ACA.

Conclusion

With young adults facing historically closed job markets, a trend that will only get worse with the global pandemic, many more are dependent on their parents for health insurance coverage and assistance with jumpstarting their careers than in the past. The racial, classed, and gendered dynamics of family obligations become an important site for researchers who hope to understand and even affect health care decision-making. Although effective family interventions are difficult to find, perhaps the simplest way to apply the lessons from this chapter is simply to make outreach and community health workers more aware of these dynamics.

For example, researchers and practitioners in Santa Ana, California, have implemented family-based health care interventions in communities with high degrees of success.[23] Their community health program recruits, trains, and engages members of Latino communities to become *"promotoras"* who can then, in turn, work to help the families within their communities better access health services. The promotoras first work on getting to know families and their dynamics, then improvise the best ways to inform, convince, and assist families with enrolling in health insurance. Their informed interventions build on local knowledge and networks and have generated higher enrollment levels.

Such community-based approaches could be significantly assisted by broader policy changes. This is where legislators could address some of the major constraints identified in this chapter. For example, Tomas's case illuminated the degradation of care work in the United States as well as the isolation of the many, many adults performing such work for their sick and disabled loved ones. Care work is racialized and gendered in both the private and public sectors, and few professional career paths provide the flexibility needed for anyone who also needs to care for disabled family members. In addition, racial and ethnic groups vary in the strength of expectations around children caring for elderly parents or grandparents. Too often, this additional work is placed on women or children in the family and comes with little or no compensation. Wealthier families are more able to pay for at-home care workers, often informally (i.e., in off-the-books arrangements) and very often by hiring low-income women, racialized people, and immigrants who lack documentation and, thus, any bargaining power.[24] When men do take on caretaking roles, it is unusual and costly in terms of personal health and career advancement—underscoring how the gendered expectations connecting women and care work have long since helped control women's autonomy.

During this study, Illinois experienced a caregiving crisis.[25] There were nowhere near enough home health aides, adult day-care programs, hospice nurses, and the like to meet the need for their labor. Even worse, a *Chicago Tribune* investigative report revealed deplorable conditions in group homes for the elderly and disabled, which had raised their prices while hiding hundreds of abuse and neglect incidents.[26] Social safety nets have a long way to go with respect to improving the most basic care needed by the chronically ill and elderly. For now, these duties generally devolve to families, especially female relatives.

That tendency is amplified among Latino families. Young adults (especially women) can be socialized to sacrifice their lives and livelihoods for the sake of their parents. For example, in households like Renee's, Latina women are often expected to clean, cook, care, and absorb emotional abuse while dismissing their pain, suffering, and health. Economic conditions solidified these social arrangements. Without the means to pay for basic necessities like food and shelter, Renee had nowhere else to go. When patriarchal family expectations operate so fiercely, it can spark a cascading array of social and emotional burdens. Children are forced to grow up fast, provide emotional support for abused parents, obey abusers, and become substitute parents to younger siblings. These dynamics sequentially, intersectionally, and cumulatively impede women's ability to acquire health insurance. They erode women's well-being and the possibility of change.

Social policy alone cannot solve the problems produced by the persistence of patriarchal family structures and norms. Feminist scholarship offers numerous perspectives for health care policymakers that emphasize the need to recognize health insurance struggles as part of economic independence struggles. Examples include efforts to promote social acceptance of more diverse family structures, gender roles, and sex roles.[27] Some scholars suggest revising policy interventions away from "saving" victims and toward removing patriarchs. Others advocate for changing representations of women by holding the media accountable for victim-blaming or privileging male-dominated perspectives. Changing societal definitions of the family, gender, and sex can help address some of the more entrenched patriarchal structures that impede women's access to benefits like health insurance.

4

The Role Gender Plays in Access to Health Care

By increasing the maximum age for a child's eligibility to remain on their parents' family health insurance plan from 23 to 26 years old, the Affordable Care Act (ACA) created a fast and easy way for parents to assist their uninsured adult children. But how does family assistance unfold for uninsured adults over 26 years old or in households where parents do not have a family health plan? These questions are relevant to many Latino households where, even in the absence of burdensome family obligations, families' assistance can unfold in deeply gendered ways. In my research, parents' expectations for their sons to serve as breadwinners produced distinct forms of family assistance for uninsured Latinos compared to Latinas. Unpacking the gendered dynamics of family assistance with securing health insurance is important for policymakers and outreach workers. Addressing the gender gap, in which Latino men are more likely to be uninsured (59%) than Latina women (41%), requires grounded knowledge of the unique challenges each group faces in the pursuit of health insurance.

In this chapter, I turn to the parents who tapped into their personal and professional networks to help their uninsured sons find health insurance through employment. Rather than inquire about the ACA or Medicaid, these families believed it was imperative that adult sons become financially independent and secure breadwinner jobs for their own future families. These families did not do the same for their daughters. The young uninsured Latina women in this study received most of their help in the form of ACA-related information conveyed by siblings or cousins who urged them to enroll by highlighting the financial consequences of remaining uninsured. Put differently, family assistance for uninsured Latino men was framed as a *quest for economic independence* but for Latina women as *averting catastrophe*.

Across my respondents, the only case in which a parent helped her adult daughter enroll in Medicaid occurred in the context of a physically abusive household. In this instance, both mother and daughter were seeking financial independence as a means of escape. Acquiring health insurance was understood as important protection on their path toward financial independence. This strategy, however, arose out of multiple failed attempts at securing protection from police, social services, and neighbors. The uninsured Latino men in this chapter received additional support from family referral networks, social workers, or labor unions, while this mother and daughter, seeking to escape abuse, tried but could not get similar institutional support.

Medicaid for Escaping an Abusive Household

"My dad broke a beer bottle over my mom's head, then bashed her head against the sharp edge of a kitchen cabinet," Camila recalled. She was 8 years old when it happened. Eleven years later, she could not recall what sparked her father's aggression.

The fear remained vivid: "I was so scared to the point where I was thinking, 'Is my dad going to kill her?' I felt so bad because I couldn't do anything about it." Camila could never understand why her father, Aurelio, was so violent. She told me that her father was always seeking complete control over her mother, Lucy; herself; and her younger siblings right up to the present.

"The other day he came home, and [my parents] started arguing. My mom was asking for respect. He went to his room and took out a condom, saying to my mom that he was going to go out and use it."

Aurelio had no college education, but he'd worked his way up to a job with good pay—enough to purchase a home and provide health insurance for the family. His wife, Lucy, a Mexican immigrant with less than a high school education, was a homemaker, and his 19-year-old daughter Camila was a college student and earned $500 a month working part-time jobs. If Aurelio ever made good on his repeated threats to leave the family and file for divorce, Camila and Lucy would be financially devastated.

The violence and threats to leave became more frequent after Camila started college. She said she believed the escalation was a symptom of his increasing insecurity—his fear that, when she attained a college degree, Camila would provide Lucy and the other kids economic independence. At random moments, without provocation, Aurelio would taunt Camila and her mother: he knew a good divorce lawyer, he reminded them, and he'd get the house if they divorced. But Camila seemed to see herself and her father recognizing the same truth: her education was the family's ticket to escape.

Camila, who had developed a passion for plants and cellular anatomy in high school, loved biology and wanted to pursue a career as a scientist. She kept her aspirations hidden from her father.

The toll of his violence both motivated the young woman's quest for economic independence and made it an ever-more overwhelming undertaking. She shouldered far more burdens and responsibilities than her peers.[1] For example, Camila served as an emotional caregiver for her mother and a substitute father for her siblings. "I have to protect them," she declared.

Often, that made her a target for her father's rage. "Every time I would intervene, try and get him off them, I would get hit."

Camila paused, wiped away a tear, and took a deep breath.

"It hurts. But I don't give up. I have to do something. I couldn't let her take it anymore. When you love your family, you don't want them to get hurt. I tell my brother and sister to hide." In the stereotypical family, parents are children's protectors. In Camila's, she saw herself as the only protection for her mother and siblings. As the oldest daughter with the most physical strength—maybe not enough to win but enough to put up a fight against a violent and often drunk grown man—Camila felt responsible to take on as much of the violence as she could. Doing otherwise, in her mind, would be shameful.

Camila and her mother grew closer as the girl grew into a teen. They would cry together, eat together, and take turns sleeping while the other kept watch for Aurelio arriving home from his regular nights out drinking. Their bond became so strong that, as Camila entered college, Lucy became more vocal in encouraging her to finish college, achieve economic independence, and help them leave their father. Together, after many attempts to get help from police and neighbors, the women determined that economic independence was the only way out.

By this time, Lucy and Aurelio were estranged from their families in Mexico. When Lucy needed help to stop Aurelio's abuse, her daughters tried going to the Chicago police department first. Even then, it had been going on for years.

"When I was 12," Camila recalled, "my little sister called the police. It was a really physical fight. My mom was bleeding pretty heavily." Camila had tried calling police, but Aurelio took the phone away. Her sister called from another room.

"The police came and my dad had the nerve to say he didn't touch her. They put him in handcuffs and took him away. My mom went to the hospital, then stayed with a neighbor. My dad spent the night in jail but came home the next day and things went back to normal."[2]

Lucy refrained from pressing charges.[3] Their neighbors provided temporary shelter for Lucy and the kids, but it was clear they couldn't offer anything permanent—nor could Chicago's scant domestic violence shelters (at the time of this study, the city had only nine domestic violence shelters serving 2.7 million residents).[4] Lucy had come face to face with the cold reality that she and her children had nowhere else to go if Aurelio ended up in prison.

Camila and her mother set their sights on achieving financial independence and decided their escape relied on Camila's education. Without Aurelio's knowledge, Lucy helped Camila fill out all the paperwork to take on thousands of dollars of student loans to pay her tuition. Rather than move into the dorms, Camila decided to continue living at home. She could commute, keep an eye on the situation with Aurelio, and save money.

* * *

In the fall of 2014, Aurelio inexplicably dropped Camila from his health insurance plan. Eligible to remain on his insurance until the age of 26, she sensed that he was either trying to undermine her or free up more cash to fund his alcohol habits. At the time, Camila worked for an on-demand, app-based valet parking service earning $11.25 an hour without insurance and saving as much money as possible.

When it came to managing her health, Camila told me she mostly counted on her immune system. When a cough or infection would not go away, she went to a neighborhood nonprofit health center recommended by a classmate. There she could pay $25 to see a nurse practitioner (another $8 or so to pick up any antibiotics they might prescribe). This was her health care safety net and, contrasting it with the doctors she saw as a child, when she was covered by her father's insurance, taught her the whole system was incredibly unequal.

At the county clinic, "[i]t was a long wait," Camila said. "I made appointments, but they were never on time. The staff were friendly, but when you look around and see that it's all people of color who are waiting, it just makes you feel inferior." That was the basis for her thinking around the ACA: "I think health insurance is a benefit only for people who can afford it," she said. "It's not available for everyone."

Camila hadn't known much about the ACA when it debuted, although she heard from the news that it financially penalized people for not having health insurance.

"Do you know how large the financial penalty is?" I asked.

"No," Camila answered.

"Then do you plan to get health insurance through the ACA?"

"I'm going to wait and see. With new things, there's always going to be problems. If other people do it and it helps them, I'll sign up. But right now, no."

Circumstances changed when Camila's mother attended a neighborhood event where ACA outreach workers shared information about Medicaid expansion. Lucy came home with a flyer, talking about how medical debt would ruin their plans to get away from Aurelio. "My mom heard at a nonprofit that I could apply for Medicaid, that it was free insurance, and so she kept badgering me to apply." After a few conversations, Camila went to the website link listed on the flyer (www.getcoveredillinois.com) and applied for Medicaid on her own.[5]

Applying for Medicaid online does not require submitting any paperwork documentation. As long as you can provide your Social Security number, the state of Illinois can verify all the information electronically or over the phone. If issues arise, a caseworker calls the applicant to request they mail in documents, but Camila's application went smoothly. Soon, she received a medical card that enabled her to visit a doctor's office in her neighborhood where, to her relief, there was little to no waiting.

"What convinced you to learn more about the ACA?" I asked.

"[My mom] kept saying that if I got into an accident, or got really sick, and ended up in the hospital, I would have to pay for it. That it would be really expensive and I would get stuck with all this debt."

"Why was your mom so insistent?" I asked.

"She knows we can't risk me getting sick and racking up all these hospital bills," said Camila. "Besides the Medicaid, she's been pushing and pushing me to get a job so we can get out and leave my dad." The two hid their plans from their abuser and worked toward starting a new life from scratch. Lucy carefully intercepted any mail related to Camila's college or Medicaid to make sure Aurelio never learned about it. She neither wanted to risk triggering a violent rage nor give Aurelio any opportunity to sabotage their plans for economic independence.

It's important to note several ways in which Camila's case differs from Renee's, in chapter 3. A similar set of interlocking social structures were at play (labor market, family, and health care), except in Camila's case, these structures operated in a way that facilitated her access to Medicaid.

Family dynamics do not always inhibit health insurance access in patriarchal households; they can also facilitate access, albeit in subversive ways.[6]

* * *

Medicaid turned out to be great for Camila, especially through her visits to a mental health clinic as the situation at home worsened. Therapy, she told me over coffee in January 2016, "is helping a lot. I learned that I have never taken the time to process all the emotional baggage from the last 20 years. I also learned I was doing the same thing my dad does: bottling up all this emotion, then taking it out on people with verbal abuse."

At the time, Camila was on academic probation. She had failed several required biology courses, and retaking them would mean getting more student loans. A student loan officer informed her she was nearing the maximum amount of money she could borrow for school and would need both parents to cosign on an additional loan if she hoped to graduate.

"I messed up." Camila sighed. She felt she'd put her careful escape plans in jeopardy, letting down her mom and siblings. "All the problems at home, the valet job, all the emotional baggage of my mom, then having to now ask my parents to cosign a loan. I feel like a failure."

The abuse at home never stopped, but Camila blamed herself for not being tough enough to weather it, work and save money, and maintain good grades.[7] She descended into a depression yet retained a sliver of hope that she could persuade her father to cosign the loan.

"I know he has problems that he just doesn't know how to deal with," Camila explained. "He just wants to drink his problems away. When he's not drunk, I try talking to him, and he just tells me I'm overly emotional, I'm a woman, and I . . . urgh! . . . it makes me so angry just thinking about it!" Medicaid was not sufficient for Camila to escape the economic conditions and abusive family dynamics that kept her trapped in this burgeoning mental health crisis, but it helped her soldier on by allowing her to access therapy.

Among other things, the counselor suggested coping mechanisms. "I started journaling to get my anger out. It's such a relief. I also joined a boxing class so I can physically get it out by punching something." Most important, Camila revealed, the appointments with the counselor had taught her that she needed to find a motivation for career success beyond just escaping her abusive father. She described it this way: "I know I need to work hard, but not just because I want to get out of a bad situation. I need to change my motivations." Beginning this journey was progress, facilitated by her mother's help enrolling in Medicaid.

The student loan conversation got put off until the fall, delayed as long as Camila could possibly delay it. And as she feared, Aurelio refused to cosign.

"He's not a big talker," Camila recalled. "He didn't give much of a reason why."

"Where do you go from here?" I asked.

"I don't have anything in mind, because I've done that before: I've planned. I've wanted things to go my way. I've envisioned futures before, and it just doesn't go my way." Camila sounded tired and resigned. "When things don't go your way, it gets really heavy."

"I'm going to try and finish college, but after that I don't know. It might be my way out, but you're always going to have a tie to your family, unless you completely drop them. I still care about [my family], even though they're broken, they don't want to change. I love them, and I want them to change, but it's a hard road. There's no painless way out. You go down kicking and screaming either way."

In my final months with Camila, she did not return to classes. Instead, she worked several jobs to try to save enough money to pay for the last semester of classes she needed to graduate. She was now working as a nanny, a valet, and a server at several restaurants, doing all the work she could find. Her Medicaid coverage protected her savings, but it was not enough to give her economic independence from Aurelio.

No aspect of the social safety net seemed equipped to help this young woman escape the patriarchal and economic structures keeping her in an abusive household. Camila's mother had, at least, managed to help her access vital health insurance benefits that were helping them survive and cope. This troubling yet powerful case shows how structural constraints and the ways they intersect are never permanent nor determinant. I left Camila with the hope that similar acts of agency exhibited by her mother as well as structural supports would ultimately help them out of their dangerous situation.

Insistent Family Members

Allison, another young Latina, had just finished her shift as a teller at a local bank when we first met to talk about the ACA. In a Logan Square Starbucks near her apartment, 22-year-old Allison described herself as a recent college graduate, uninsured, and struggling to find better-paying work. She said that she liked President Obama (primarily because of the way he treated his wife, Michelle), but she did not have much enthusiasm for the ACA.

"Do you think the ACA will help you?" I asked.

"Maybe, I don't know what it will get me into. There are probably things it won't cover, but it might be better than nothing." When it came to the ACA, Allison was not an optimist. She based her assessment on an experience with the county health care system just the year before.

Shortly after becoming uninsured (when her father lost his job), Allison started experiencing debilitating back pain. She could barely move without having excruciating pain and her condition was not improving. Needing to work and attend classes, Allison visited the Cook County hospital emergency room for help.

"I waited three hours to meet with a doctor who just asked me a few questions and gave me some prescription pain medicine," said Allison. The pain medicine helped, and her back pain subsided, but a few weeks later, she received a bill in the mail: $350. "I knew I'd get a bill," Allison allowed, "but I didn't know it would be that much for a 15-minute talk with a doctor and some pills. Now, I think twice about whether I should go to the emergency room or see a doctor for something."

Allison's sister Teresa worked at a neighborhood health clinic in Logan Square. When all three of us met up in the winter of 2014, Teresa reprimanded and counseled her sister on seeking out health care.

"The emergency room is the worst possible place you could have gone!" said Teresa.

"I didn't know!" Allison retorted.

"You should have gone to my clinic; they have money set aside for people without insurance. We could have got you those pain meds for a lot cheaper!" Teresa pivoted, telling Allison, "You know, you should apply for Obamacare. You'll probably qualify because of your age and income. I don't sign people up, but I know the navigator who does at our clinic."

"Yeah, I don't know." Allison hesitated, adding, "I'll wait and see."

"What is there to 'wait and see'?" Teresa asked with a raised voice. "You're lucky it wasn't more than $350."

"OK, I'll think about [it]." Allison changed the topic of conversation.

* * *

A year later, we met again at the very same coffee shop. This time, Allison told me she was enrolled in Medicaid.

"What happened?" I asked about her change of heart.

"Basically, my sister scared me into applying."

"Oh yeah?"

"Yeah, she kept on telling me that if I had a medical emergency or got into a bad car accident, the medical bills would put me in debt for the rest of my life." Allison vividly recalled Teresa's nagging: "What if something happens? You're going to have all this debt!" With the help of the health navigator at the clinic where her sister worked, Allison finally enrolled.

Allison's family member had an enabling role in helping her secure insurance, warning her of potentially dire outcomes if she remained uninsured. This was a pattern I saw among a number of Latina Medicaid enrollees.

Six months after enrolling in Medicaid, however, Allison had only used it a few times, to get physicals or immunizations required for work. This was despite having caught a flu and continuing to experience recurrences of her terrible back pain. She hesitated to use her Medicaid for doctor's visits or any other form of care, because the memory of that unexpected $350 ER bill loomed large.

"Why haven't you visited a doctor about your back?" I asked.

"You never know what's going to happen," she answered, "or what expenses might come up. Mainly, having health insurance has given me peace of mind that if I get seriously sick, like in a hospital for a long time, that I'll have some financial protection, but I still avoid using it if I can."

Allison still viewed the health care safety net as a resource of last resort—and she didn't count her back pain or flu as being "seriously sick." She relied more on self-medicating and advice from friends, even though she now had Medicaid. We can see here that it is crucial to separate *health insurance coverage* from *health care usage*. The forces shaping one may not be the same ones or operate in the same way, shaping the usage of health care benefits.

I followed up with Allison for the final time in 2016. She had moved to Philadelphia for a job as an administrator at a community college, but her new state had not expanded Medicaid eligibility under the ACA. Her only option there was to purchase private health insurance on the ACA exchange or go uninsured. At the same time, her father landed a new job in Chicago, and so he added her to his new health insurance plan. This strategy of enrolling in a parent's health insurance plan turned out to be a common alternative to the ACA for uninsured Latino millennials, especially men.

Family Referrals

"My personal ambition has always been to help people. It may sound silly, but I think that's my whole purpose in life. Since I was a kid, I volunteered at a lot of nonprofits and have been involved in numerous grassroots efforts to improve the community." Earnestly, 27-year-old Ramon Lozano described his experience as the first in his working-class family to attend college. He had earned a degree in political science from a local university, but unable to find work, he was still living with his parents in Logan Square. He thought pursuing a master's degree might boost his job prospects, although the tuition put that option out of reach for the time being.

Ramon's father worked at a factory, and his mother worked at a fast-food restaurant. He contributed his income as a part-time server at a restaurant, and together, the family's combined household income enabled them to care for Ramon's elderly grandmother.

For most of his life, Ramon had been insured through his father's health insurance plan. That had changed recently: "My father had to stop working because of a degenerative kidney disease. It weakened him so much that it prevented him from working. He had to quit his job and be placed on a transplant list." The hospital helped Ramon's father enroll in disability benefits and Medicaid, but Ramon was no longer insured at this point in 2013.

The young man told me he was unsure whether he would seek out information about the newly enacted ACA. He did not have any memorable past experiences (positive or negative) with the health care safety net, telling me he stayed informed about the new policy when it was covered by local and national news sources. Nonetheless, Ramon was still unaware that he was now eligible for Medicaid. He was going to wait a bit longer before inquiring about the ACA, focusing on applying for jobs that might provide health insurance.

* * *

Within six months, Ramon had enrolled in Medicaid. The process of getting Ramon's father on disability required multiple meetings with a social worker. At one of those meetings, Ramon's grandmother mentioned that her grandson was uninsured, and the social worker, in turn, brought up the likelihood that he was eligible for Medicaid. Back at home, Ramon's grandmother relayed that information, and he attended the next meeting with the social worker.

Enrolling "was pretty easy," Ramon remembered, saying the social worker "walked me through everything on her laptop." He "got a medical card in the mail a month later."

Like the others in this chapter, Ramon's family facilitated his Medicaid enrollment. While he was dependent on his family for financial support, however, Ramon was not constrained by structures of patriarchy or negative past experiences with the county health care system. He did not share other respondents' sense of urgency regarding being uninsured, and he was not fearful of interacting with the health care safety net.

Ramon's case further illuminates how families can be key sites of information sharing and building policy intelligence with respect to health insurance. Family members with network ties to social workers, health navigators, or promotoras can become further ambassadors, helping their fellow family members through the complexities of the health care system and addressing their concerns.

Now insured, Ramon said of Medicaid, "I'm glad it's there so that I don't get stuck with a huge bill if I get hit by a bus or something. But the main thing I'm trying to do is find a job in politics or public policy that's more in line with what I want to do. I don't plan on being on this [Medicaid] for too long." He saw the safety net as helpful and temporary—a way to get through a tough time.

In my final correspondence with Ramon in 2015, he found a job in the restaurant industry that provided health insurance benefits. It was at a high-end restaurant in one of Chicago's more affluent neighborhoods, a job he applied for solely because of the better pay and benefits. This was good news, yet Ramon felt his prospects of finding a job in politics or public policy slipping away.

"Many of the entry-level jobs in politics or public policy don't provide benefits, and they don't pay well." Ramon thought, "Unless you have a graduate degree or political connections, you can't find a good job, so I'm kind of stuck in this job now because of its pay and benefits. If I leave to pursue the work I really want to do, I give that up, and right now, I can't afford to give it up."

"How much do those entry-level jobs pay?"

"It's not terrible," Ramon said, "the problem is that you earn too much to be eligible for Medicaid, and if I were to buy a health insurance plan through the ACA it would come with a deductible between $1,000 to $6,000. That means that if I get sick, I have to pay the first $1,000, and I just don't have the money in my savings to survive that." With bleak job prospects and a relatively good understanding of the differences between types of health coverage, Ramon joined many of the other Latino millennials in this study who appeared stuck in an uncertain position of waiting for the next opportunity to come.

Financial Independence for Men

An aspiring DJ with a passion for music and the arts, 25-year-old Raymundo Lopez held an associate's degree from community college and felt ready to pursue a full-time music career. "I don't have enough money or training to produce music digitally," said Raymundo. "I mostly use analog and cheap music production software." Nonetheless, he produced numerous tracks on free internet platforms, played live shows, and posted videos of his performances on social media, working on establishing his reputation and eventually his financial independence.

For the time being, he lived in the same Little Village house he grew up in, supported in his ambitions by his parents. His mother worked as the principal of an elementary school, a job with health insurance benefits that would cover Raymundo until he turned 26. In our first interview, Raymundo expressed no interest in politics, government, or the news, and he told me he had no opinion of the ACA or the health care safety net.

In our follow-up a year later, Raymundo was 25 and feeling his mother's pressure to reconsider his career options. "She told me I was going to get kicked off her health insurance plan when I turn 26," Raymundo recalled, "and that I needed some kind of job that was going to get me insurance." Raymundo didn't think it was that big of a deal because he never had major health problems or emergencies, but dependent on his parents, he went along with his mom's advice.

Searching for jobs online and through friendship networks, Raymundo said, "The only full-time job openings I found that pay decent [and have insurance] were to be cops and firefighters, and I don't want to do either of those."

Raymundo's mother stepped in and used her professional networks to find him a part-time job at a nearby high school. It didn't pay much, although she believed it could lead to a full-time position with health insurance benefits. "I wouldn't mind helping out and teaching kids music or arts," Raymundo commented. And after another year, the strategy had paid off: Raymundo was now a full-time arts teacher at the high school, and his job came with health insurance benefits.

As we caught up over lunch, Raymundo shared funny stories of adjusting to his role as an educator and adult-in-charge: "I'm not that much older than the kids," Raymundo said, "so when they say funny inappropriate stuff to me in Spanish during class, I have to try hard to not laugh."

He was still producing music and performing DJ sets, but much less frequently since teaching required him to be awake and out the door by 6:30 a.m.—not a great fit for the late-night party and club scene. During our final interview in late 2016, he was still happy, a working arts teacher and insured.

In contrast to so many of my respondents, Raymundo's life was pretty calm and uneventful during the three years of this study. His mother and the help she provided were critical in this respect. Raymundo had consistent stable financial and social support from his parents. When he was on the brink of losing health insurance coverage, his mother not only anticipated this, but she also found him an opportunity to get both health insurance and a stable income. As a result, Raymundo never even had to entertain the scenario of enrolling in Medicaid.

* * *

Family job referral networks were similarly important for Oliver Klozov, a 23-year-old Mexican American who had been uninsured for three years when I first met him in 2013. Like Raymundo, Oliver was insured through his parents' family plan, but like Ramon, he'd suddenly became uninsured when his father lost his job. At the time, Oliver was 20 and worked for a company selling cell phones in shopping malls. The job brought in just over $20,000 a year, enough to allow Oliver to afford an apartment with roommates but not enough to afford insurance (and possibly too much to qualify for Medicaid, had the ACA expansion been in place at the time).

At a family party, Oliver talked about his health insurance situation with his uncle who worked as a plumber. In Chicago, plumbers are unionized, working as "journeymen" (individuals who work on-call) or for plumbing contractors for specific jobs like new building construction. Through their union's affiliation with the National United Association of Plumbers and Pipefitters, Chicago-area plumbers earn $47.50 an hour with full health insurance, dental, and vision benefits. They are trained and certified directly by the union, and applicants only need to have a high school diploma. Of course, Oliver's uncle pointed out, this meant there were far more applicants than jobs, and it could take years to even learn the outcome of your application. Still, he encouraged Oliver to at least apply. It wasn't his preferred career, but it offered the stability and financial independence becoming so scarce in the US job market. "I didn't expect to get a call back," Oliver explained, and he didn't.

Six months after our first interview, Oliver accepted a promotion from his cell phone company. It didn't come with insurance, although the higher pay and lower cost of living enticed him to take the new position in Phoenix, Arizona. Although Arizona was a Medicaid expansion state, Oliver had very little knowledge of the ACA or Medicaid.

"I'm not holding my breath for free health insurance," Oliver said about the ACA. "All I've heard is that the Republicans have tried 40 times to kill it, so I don't even know if it's going to be around much longer."

"Then what do you do when you get sick?" I asked.

"I try natural remedies or I'll just go to the gym and try to sweat it out."

He shared that, a few months after moving to Phoenix, his tonsils had become severely swollen. "I came to work anyway, and my co-workers were like, 'You got to go to the doctor.' But I told them I don't have health insurance. The swelling got so bad that my boss ordered me to the hospital. So, I found some free clinic on the web. They still charged me, but it wasn't bad. $99 for the visit and $300 dollars for them to drain my tonsils and [get me] some antibiotics."

Oliver brought up that, sure, living uninsured in Phoenix was hard, but it was nothing compared to the hardship of living as a Mexican American in Phoenix.

"They're really anti-immigration out here," Oliver said over the phone. "Like 15 of my friends have been pulled over by police who just ask them for ID. I've only been pulled over once, but it's crazy. You see ICE [Immigration and Customs Enforcement] around here a lot, too."

The combination of poor health care, anti-Latino sentiment, and hot weather pushed Oliver to move back to Chicago. He didn't have a job lined up.

One week after Oliver moved back into his parents' house, that union application his uncle had urged him to put in suddenly reappeared. The plumber's union called: they accepted his application and were ready to enroll him in their trade school. Oliver wasn't thrilled about becoming a plumber, but he was definitely thrilled to have landed a stable job with a good income and great health insurance benefits. "They cover 90% of everything," Oliver enthused of the insurance benefits, "and they put a portion of my check into a fund for me to pay for whatever expenses I have out of pocket, so I end paying very little. I've never had health insurance this good. Ever." For the first time in more than five years, Oliver went to the dentist.

For our final interview, in the fall of 2016, I met Oliver near a downtown Chicago construction site. Part of a team installing a new sewage system, Oliver left his hard hat on as he sipped coffee with me at a shop nearby. He seemed proud to tell me that he'd purchased a home in a suburb and a new car to commute. Like Raymundo, Oliver's family support had helped him acquire income stability and health insurance through employment that might not have been their dream jobs but looked like sure paths to upward mobility.

* * *

Newt McCarthy was a heavyset 29-year-old white man who originally attempted to join the Marines straight out of high school. When he could not pass the physical fitness test required for boot camp, he settled for two years of community college and an associate's degree. By the time we sat down for our first extended conversation over a diner breakfast, Newt had been working as a security guard for eight years. He lived in Logan Square with his mother and siblings.

Newt had identified with his father, a politically conservative former Marine who worked as a police officer in the city. They used to watch Fox News together. In 2012, Newt's father died by suicide, leaving his family devastated and on the verge of an economic crisis.

"What happened with my father put me, as the oldest son, in the position of having to pay the majority of the bills," said Newt, adding, "My mother pays a lot of the bills too. My brother works, but my sister doesn't have a job. We're basically living paycheck to paycheck." It had only been about a year, and Newt shared, "I can't really say what the future holds for us."

The ACA and Medicaid held the potential to significantly benefit Newt and help address his economic precarity and uninsurance. But he staunchly opposed the ACA on political grounds and told me the policy was perilous for society as a whole.

"Look, there is nothing wrong with trying to make sure people are healthy and all that," he began. "But if hardworking people are paying for their own health insurance, why make it free for everyone else? The health insurance I'd get from the ACA is not 'free,' because I'd be getting it from tax revenue from other people paying into the system." Newt was disinclined to benefit from an unjust transfer of wealth from the rich to the poor, although he knew his family's situation needed to improve. If things continued as they were, it would only be a matter of time before they would be forced to depend on the state for medical care.

Newt started making phone calls to his father's old co-workers. "I never wanted to become a police officer," said Newt, "but it's an option I always knew I had because of my dad and all his friends."

As a 15-year veteran of the Chicago Police Department, Newt's father had befriended dozens of officers from jurisdictions all over Cook County. Tapping into this network, Newt was sure he didn't want to work in Chicago. Thus, he focused on making calls to family friends who could provide inside help on landing a job as a police officer in a suburban jurisdiction. After a few months, Newt was called to interview for three different suburban police departments. He accepted a position an hour west of Chicago (although it allowed Newt to continue living in the city with his family). The starting salary was $60,000 per year with full health insurance benefits. After 30 years on the job, he could retire at age 60 with a lifetime pension.

Like Raymundo and Oliver, Newt relied on family networks to get an inside track to a job with health insurance benefits. He was able to avert the need to interact with the ACA. Newt and I met for a final time in 2016 in the western suburbs where he now worked. Newt's political beliefs had not changed, and he was happy with the health insurance and financial stability provided by his job.

Altering Gendered Pathways to Health Insurance

Family assistance for Latino men took on the form of help with job-seeking whereas, for Latina women, it took on the form of information sharing and referrals to social services. Because jobs providing health insurance benefits have grown scarce, the difference may explain why Latina women are now less likely to be uninsured than Latino men. Qualitative studies of Latino men have added an attitudinal dimension, in that they reveal a tendency to perceive social services as feminized and, therefore, more appropriate for women than for themselves.[8]

To date, community-based interventions aimed at improving health care access for Latinos have tapped into the family networks of grandparents, siblings, cousins, aunts, and uncles who connect uninsured Latinos to social workers or health navigators that might provide health insurance.[9] Advancing this work, particularly for Latino men, might involve focusing on employers or workplaces as potential sites of recruitment or health care outreach. This strategy, however, can only be effective if more Latino men can help transform the feminized meaning of seeking assistance.

Camila's story of enrolling in Medicaid despite the awful constraints of an abusive household illuminates both the power of women's agency and resilience and the woefully inadequate institutional support for domestic violence survivors. Domestic violence sparks a cascading array of social and emotional burdens. Children are forced to grow up fast or, like Camila, take on the role of emotional caretaker for an abused parent and substitute parent for younger siblings. Although the ACA expanded funding for clinics to conduct domestic violence screening, this would have made little difference for Camila or Renee, who rarely went to clinics and did not have the economic independence to exit their situations. The ACA alone, quite simply, cannot solve the problem of domestic violence. Other societal institutions like the family, police, and schools also require reform if policymakers and advocates are serious about helping women and children escape dangerous situations (let alone ending domestic violence).

One underexplored strategy for assisting uninsured Latinas would be to work toward improving their access to the kinds of jobs that provide health insurance benefits. Police, plumbing, restaurant work, and public education were the labor market sectors that the Latino men in this chapter entered to acquire health insurance benefits. It's also worth noting that labor unions play a key role for workers in each of these sectors, especially in Chicago. This suggests that supporting labor unions (which organize to secure and protect worker health insurance benefits) and helping Latinos enter firmly unionized professions (like policing and firefighting) in which they are historically underrepresented would be good ways to advance their health insurance enrollment.

5

The Power of Social Networks to Secure Insurance

Dozens of Latino health care professionals packed a seventh-floor conference room in Chicago's Merchandise Mart to discuss strategies for enrolling low-income uninsured Latinos in health insurance plans. Alonzo, the director of a nonprofit organization, presented his strategy of targeting the college-aged Latino population. "Health insurance is not the most exciting issue," he said emphatically to the audience with a PowerPoint slide clicker in hand. "But you all have heard of the 'Got Milk?' campaign?" The ads he referenced were a campaign originally designed in 1993 for a California-based industry group, and they famously featured celebrities posing with "milk mustaches" on their upper lips. Magazine spreads and billboards across the country were soon asking "Got Milk?"

"Check this out!" Alonzo exclaimed as his power-point slide came up on the screen (see figure 5.1). Alonzo's campaign idea borrowed from the "Brosurance" ad campaign created by the Colorado Consumer Health Initiative, which replaced the question mark from the "Got milk?" campaign with an exclamation point: "Got Insurance!" In it, a young man slings his arm around Uncle Sam, toasting his insurance coverage with red Solo cups over a beer keg. "Party on!" Alonzo yelled, trying to get the crowd in on the fun, but no one laughed.

This particular outreach idea didn't resonate, although it demonstrated the group's awareness that, with half of uninsured Latinos between the ages of 18 and 35, college campuses would be important Affordable Care Act (ACA) outreach sites. Because college students tend to be younger, healthier, and less likely than other groups to view health insurance as an immediate need, some policymakers refer to them as the "young and invincible" population—a group stubbornly unwilling to imagine they will become seriously ill and need health insurance.[1]

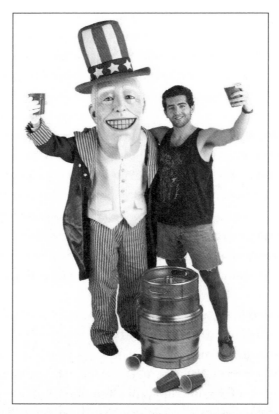

FIGURE 5.1. ACA College Outreach Flyer. Source:
Ad created by the Colorado Consumer Health
Initiative.

College-aged students in the United States often only begin to consider acquiring health insurance when a serious unanticipated health crisis arises, at which point the process of seeking health insurance is especially urgent and stressful. For some, the failure to quickly resolve a health crisis can lead to more physical pain and financial suffering, cascading into other crises. Outreach workers understood that it would be hard to convince the uninsured college-aged Latinos and African Americans in this chapter with ads positioning insurance as fun, exciting, or a must-have accessory. Instead, they looked to the interpersonal and inter-institutional networks provided by campus life to boost awareness of their eligibility for health insurance and smooth access to enrolling. Sociologist Mario Small refers to the idea on which this strategy rests as "organizational embeddedness," capturing the network advantages that organizations create for people in unexpected and unanticipated ways.[2]

When faced with a health crisis, the respondents in this chapter relied heavily on their classmates as they sought out information about applying for health insurance through the ACA. Their college referral networks played a mundane yet powerful role in helping young uninsured Latino and African American adults acquire coverage, and they suggest that other institutional locations where young uninsured adults live, work, or visit during a health crisis can be seeded with simple, straightforward information and resources to boost outreach programs. The information conveyed through social networks at college helped the uninsured Latinos in my study overcome the anxieties about the health care safety net produced from negative past experiences, revealing another structural nexus shaping insurance access.

Getting a Flyer from a Classmate

Dressed in a shirt, tie, and red vest, Alan (a 28-year-old African American man) sat at a large poker table, dealing cards to the 11 players seated around him. There were 30 more tables like his, each with a teacher or school administrator dealing cards at the South Side Charter charity poker tournament. Alan taught English at the high school, which predominantly served low-income black youth. Since the 1990s, charter schools have blossomed throughout Chicago, and Alan liked teaching at South Side. But charter school staff are not members of the Chicago teachers' union and, thus, are paid far less than traditional public school teachers. To improve his employment prospects, Alan quit his job at South Side Charter (which did provide health insurance) and enrolled in a master's degree program full-time. He was uninsured when the ACA rolled out in 2013.

A number of past experiences left Alan skeptical about the ACA. He told me about one student at South Side, a severely overweight kid who complained of chest pains. Alan worried the student was experiencing a heart attack and, when the school day ended, drove the young man to the nearest emergency room. For three tense hours, Alan recalled, "I'm sitting there with him, trying to flag down a nurse to tell them he's having serious chest pain, but no one came. It was like no one cared." The student's mother eventually arrived, thanked Alan, and told him he could go home. Alan wished them well and left. To this day, he's not sure how long the student waited or what diagnosis he was given. The student never came back to school.

The experience reinforced Alan's lack of faith in county health care facilities. His memorable personal experience occurred when he was 17, living in his small Indiana hometown. Alan's family frequented county hospitals and clinics for health care, and so, when his mother started vomiting blood, she saw a specialist at the public hospital. "Oh, I think you just have a bad case of gas," he remembered the first doctor telling his mother. It would take three more visits to specialists before she was properly diagnosed—and learned she needed emergency surgery. Musing aloud, Alan asked me, "Is that a reflection on all public hospitals? I don't want to say, but there was a series of doctors who told her she just had bad gas, and I'm not going to bet my health on that kind of medical treatment."

Thankfully, Alan's mother recovered, but these experiences led Alan to believe that safety net programs did not provide access to high-quality health care. That could come only through securing a "good" job. In the meantime, as an uninsured graduate student, Alan googled symptoms when he got sick and tried out home remedies to relieve them. He changed his exercise habits, in order to do workouts that came with less risk of serious injury. And he hoped for the best.

"Do you think the ACA will help you?" I asked.

"I'm not holding my breath," said Alan. "I've learned not to expect much, but I hope it will."

"What's the basis of your hope?"

"My hope for a better America, one that cares about each person. I know I sound like Obama when I say that," he said cheekily. Alan wanted his preconceptions proved wrong when it came to the health care overhaul. In large part, his hope drew on his strong Christian faith. Raised in a churchgoing family, faith and hope had always played a large role in Alan's life.

Six months later, he was still uninsured, but with faith and hope, he scheduled an appointment with a health navigator at a county health clinic in his neighborhood to simply gather more information about the ACA. He doubted that the ACA could help him but figured that going to the county clinic seeking more *information* was unlikely to hurt. He was wrong.

* * *

"Hello, I have a 4:30 p.m. appointment with a health navigator," Alan said, greeting the receptionist. The West Side Health Clinic, where Alan booked his appointment, served a predominantly black low-income clientele in the North Lawndale neighborhood. That day, the clinic was empty. The only sound in the waiting, fingers on her keyboard.

We waited just a few minutes until Tiffany, an African American health navigator led us to a large room filled with cubicles. Each station had a desktop computer.

"You can sit right there," said Tiffany to Alan as she pointed to one of the little desks.

"Thanks," Alan answered. "I have a few questions."

"OK, you don't want to apply?" Tiffany said in confusion.

"Not today," Alan clarified. "I want to know what I'm applying for before I sign up."

"OK, are you employed?"

"I don't even know how to answer that question," Alan answered with embarrassment. As a graduate student, Alan had a job working at the university, but it was compensated in tuition reductions rather than pay-checks. He began, "I work at a place where I don't get paid for but. . . ."

Tiffany interrupted. "Then you are not employed."

I could see that the words landed like a gut punch. Alan hadn't ex-pected the navigator to be so blunt.

She continued. "If you are not employed, you are going to qualify for [a] medical card with Medicaid. With Medicaid you can go anywhere and do anything. It covers medical and vision."

"OK," Alan replied.

Tiffany could not sense that Alan felt overwhelmed by the rapid-fire information. So she kept going. "Medicaid is like Blue Cross/Blue Shield, because you can do anything and everything with it." By referring to a well-recognized insurance brand, Tiffany sought a shorthand compari-son for Medicaid benefits.

Instead, Alan admitted, "I've never had health insurance since I've lived in Chicago, so I don't even know what that means."

The navigator ignored his comment, reaching for two small forms on the desk. "Can I get both of you to sign these cards?" she asked, indicat-ing both Alan and myself. "We're not going to call you. I just need your name and address to say that I talked to you. That is all, OK?" I under-stood that the state government, in an effort to evaluate health navigator performance, required everyone with whom they interacted to fill out a form. The form helped produce metrics about the number of people navigators assisted.

In the meantime, Alan asked directly, "Why do you need our infor-mation?" Since he was just there to gather information, it was a fair question.

Tiffany replied sarcastically, her voice slowed and dripping with con-descension: "To . . . say . . . that . . . I . . . talked . . . to . . . you. . . ." After a beat, she added, "I mean, you're not signing anything; you are just putting your name, address, and phone number. That is how we keep up with who we talk to and who we track." That last phrase was a poor choice of words. By saying "who we track," Tiffany contradicted her earlier statement that the information served no purpose. And the idea of being tracked tends to put most people on edge.

It certainly discomforted Alan. He put down the form and tried to get back to the purpose of his visit. "I just came here to get more information," Alan repeated. "If I sign up, what do I get?"

"Health insurance, which is medical and vision."

"Right, but there's *good* insurance and *bad* insurance," Alan remarked. "How do I know if Medicaid is good or bad?"

"It's good. That's why I compared it to Blue Cross/Blue Shield."

"But what does that *mean*?" Alan asked in frustration.

"It covers everything and, visually, you can get glasses."

Alan leaned back in his chair as if to collect his thoughts. Before he could be convinced to sign up for anything, Alan wanted to see what plans were available, pick up a pamphlet, or look at options on a website. He certainly wanted more than Tiffany's word.

"OK, well, is there anything else I should know because, coming in, I didn't think Medicaid was the only option for me," Alan explained. "I do work. I actually work at a local university. But they pay me to go to school."

Tiffany was, by now, frustrated as well, and she raised her voice: "Exactly, so you are unemployed."

Alan knew that Medicaid was an insurance program for low-income people. He didn't know if it cost anything, where specifically he could use it, and whether it was high quality. To him, it conjured memories of watching his mother suffer while doctors dismissed her pain, of his student waiting hours with potentially serious chest pains before he could access "emergency" medical care.

None of Tiffany's words did anything to open up a conversation that would have helped her understand, let alone address, Alan's concerns. Instead, Tiffany made Alan feel dumb for asking questions and hesitating to apply. Moreover, by sharply and repeatedly informing Alan he was, in her eyes at least, unemployed, she reinforced the stigma of public aid and amplified his sense that Medicaid was low-quality health care for poor people, a last resort.

By the time Tiffany finally began to explain the ACA's Medicaid expansion, Alan had already checked out of the conversation. "Usually Medicaid was for pregnant women, kids, the disabled," Tiffany explained, "but now that Obama has passed this, it helps people like you who are going to school and not working."

He was done. "OK, cool," deflected Alan. "This took me in a whole other direction than I thought. I don't have any more questions." He stood up to leave, and again Tiffany insisted, "Wait, you guys still have to fill these forms." Alan grabbed a pen and filled it out. (Later, he'd share that he hadn't provided his real information on the form.)

As we walked toward the nearest train station, Alan erupted, "Man, she was pushy!"

"Yeah," I confirmed.

"She was like, 'Well, if you don't have insurance, you need insurance.' In my head, I was thinking, 'I know!' I didn't know how to even ask questions after that." He shook his head, "She kept on talking about Blue Cross/Blue Shield, but I didn't know what that meant." Alan couldn't stop thinking about the encounter, even after we boarded the train. It was starting down the tracks as Alan commented, "I think she was being presumptuous. Like, she thought we were these poor unemployed dudes and that we could just be told to fill out an application." To me, this seemed like it was going to be the third strike against Alan getting insured.

* * *

Six months later, Alan was still uninsured but on track to graduating on time and still hopeful his master's degree would open up a field of jobs with health insurance benefits. His plan was working smoothly until he contracted a nagging cough. As it worsened, Alan cycled through home remedies: herbs, tea, cough lozenges, a humidifier. Nothing worked, so he began canvassing his classmates for ideas.

"A classmate of mine gave me this recipe to blend crushed tomatoes, ginger, jalapenos, onions, and some other stuff," said Alan with a frown. "I drank it. It didn't work. It was disgusting."

His cough was loud, dry, and hoarse. After weeks, it started interfering with his coursework. Alan would sit near the classroom door so he could quickly exit the room when his cough acted up during lectures. He stopped exercising because the heavy breathing made his cough worse. Worst of all, he was miserable, getting just two or three hours of sleep a night. "I had a 20-page paper due at the end of the semester," said Alan, "and I just couldn't focus." Simply walking to and from the train and class was taxing, and no matter how many home remedies his fellow students offered up, he was still sick—and $150 poorer, having spent all his discretionary cash on his attempts.

Near the end of the semester, one of his classmates shared a flyer that contained information about the ACA. "I remember the ad saying you can apply by yourself online," Alan said, perhaps thinking of Tiffany. "So I just did." He saw the ACA as a last resort, and with empty pockets and a mysterious cough, well, it was time for the last resort.

In a follow-up interview at a coffee shop, Alan recounted enrolling using his laptop. Although ACA websites had highly publicized problems, by December 2014, many of the glitches had been fixed. So Alan navigated to the healthcare.gov website, where a window popped up with two options: (1) see if I can enroll and (2) see if I can change. He clicked on "see if I can enroll" and another window popped open, asking for his zip code. Alan entered the information and was redirected to Illinois's state ACA enrollment website, getcoveredillinois.gov.

There, he recalled, Alan answered a series of questions to determine whether he should apply for Medicaid or shop for health insurance plans on the Illinois marketplace. Entering information like his average monthly income, household size, and age, Alan quickly learned he could be eligible for Medicaid, then clicked on a box that read "start my Medicaid application." This took him to abe.illinois.gov, the same official website Illinois's social workers, health navigators, and health care personnel used to enroll the uninsured.

This website required Alan to create a username and password and then asked simply whether he would like to apply for "healthcare." It's worth noting that the website didn't use the name of specific programs like Medicaid, in favor of more vague terms like *health care*. This seemed to help reduce the confusion as, in Alan's mind, he was just applying for health care. Now the site informed Alan to gather some information for his application, including his Social Security number, mailing address, and his full name and date of birth.

Moving ahead, the site prompted Alan to answer whether he would additionally like to apply for cash assistance or food stamps—the same "bundling" innovation introduced by the Illinois Department of Health and Family Services that helped Sandra, in chapter 2, access multiple forms of assistance and get back on her feet. Alan declined and continued to entering information everyone living in his household. He listed the names and birth dates of his roommates.

Now the site moved on to income.

The prompt asked, "How often does Alan get paid, and how much does Alan get paid each time they are paid?"

As Alan's job helped pay off his tuition, and as he was taking out student loans to pay for his living expenses, he entered $0 (if nothing else, Tiffany had likely impressed on him that, to the government, he was considered unemployed). Did Alan have any other income sources such as from other government programs, retirement accounts, or from friends and family, asked the site. And finally, he was asked to estimate his expenses, specifically, child support, spousal support payments, medical bills, or other bills.

When he got to the final page, Alan was asked to review all his information and then check a box indicating that he had read and understood the "fraud affidavit penalty." It read: "I understand that the information on this form is subject to verification by federal, state, and local officials. If I intentionally give false or misleading information, I may be subject to criminal or civil prosecution." The warning, which all applicants must attest to, said nothing of what those criminal or civil penalties might be (a fact that may dissuade some people who are particularly concerned about potential interactions with criminal justice actors). Alan nevertheless checked the box, electronically signed the application, and clicked "submit."

As the final confirmation indicated, Alan did receive a phone call from what he called "a social worker," following up to confirm his Social Security number, address, and employment at the university. Two weeks after that, Alan received an insurance card. He was officially enrolled in Medicaid.

"What got you to apply?" I asked.

"I was desperate," Alan recalled. Without health care to handle his cough, he added, "I was afraid I was going to fail one of my classes."

In the weeks he waited to hear the outcome of his Medicaid application, Alan conducted a Google search for the nearest doctor who would see him. Going to the clinic, he learned that his cough was a form of bronchitis triggered by allergies. Subsequent testing revealed at least a dozen allergies, and the doctor prescribed Alan several anti-allergy medications. He felt better within days. Alan convinced his professor to grant an extension for his 20-page paper, which he turned in on time (it ended up being the only B Alan received while in graduate school). In a text message, Alan told me happily, "I can breathe again; I can sleep again!"

Alan even found the staff at the doctor's office helpful. They asked for a copy of his Medicaid application and used that to send his bill directly to the state. After his trio of bad experiences, this positive story of seeking and receiving medical care that helped quickly and integrated with his Medicaid even while it was pending was a big change for Alan.

"I expected a large bill but was pleasantly surprised to see it covered everything. Even the prescription medications." It had taken a severe illness and a classmate referral to get Alan on Medicaid, and I wondered whether he might have avoided all that suffering and the drop in his school performance if his appointment with Tiffany the health navigator had gone better.

* * *

When I followed up with Alan a year later, he had earned his master's degree and was working as a college counselor at a local university. The job provided good pay, and rather than Medicaid, he was now enrolled in his employer's health insurance plan. His positive experience with Medicaid and the ACA had changed his perceptions of the health care safety net for the better.

"The experience taught me to be more responsible about health insurance," Alan said, "to not just assume it's all bad and avoid it, but to do serious research on it. Learn the details and be more persistent." In hindsight, Alan felt he should have sought help elsewhere after his unhelpful interaction with Tiffany. He attributed his lack of persistence to immaturity—and a young man's tendency to think himself invincible.

"It taught me that you have to be 'benefit-savvy,'" Alan explained. "That by itself is a benefit the ACA has given me. It's given me a life lesson: government benefits are good, but government bureaucracy . . . not so much." In this answer, Alan indicated a distinction between government benefits and the sometimes flawed frontline bureaucrats in charge of administering those benefits.

Alan's experience with the ACA, eventually brokered through a seemingly mundane act—a flyer thrust into his hand by a concerned classmate—redefined his relationship with the health care safety net. It taught him the importance of patience, persistence, and thick skin. In his words, it made him more "benefit-savvy." And very likely, in his new position as a college counselor on a university campus, that experience was translated into proactive policy knowledge shared with more and more students.

Info from College Roommate

Twenty-two-year-old Anita Montes was a Latina who spent most of her life in Detroit. She'd had more than her fair share of encounters with a broken safety net. When she was just 10 years old, her mother had a heart attack and died. Anita's father and older brother were her primary caretakers in those tough times. "We lived paycheck to paycheck on my dad's salary as a plumber," said Anita. "All the money went to rent, utilities, and food. We really didn't have extra money for anything else."

Most of Anita's subsequent experience with the health care safety net came from caring for other family members. For instance, during her freshman year of high school, her father had a stroke that paralyzed the left side of his body. She and her brother were panicked, she remembered. "We didn't have any savings to hold us over."

"While he was in the hospital, my brother and I tried to get him disability benefits," but the application was tough, and it got rejected anyway. Anita turned to the pastor at their church for help, and he referred her to a lawyer in their congregation who helped the siblings appeal the disability denial at no charge. It turned out that Anita and her brother did not provide enough detail on how the stroke prevented their father from continuing work. One year later, Anita resubmitted the paperwork, completed an in-person interview, and the state overturned its decision.

The disability checks started coming in, although at just $700 a month, it was nowhere near enough to make ends meet. With the guidance of their now-disabled father, Anita and her brother generated income informally by doing small plumbing jobs for friends and neighbors. Their father would instruct them on what to do and which tools to use, and Anita and her brother would do the physical work. The family got by, but it was always a close call.

The experience navigating the safety net on her father's behalf shaped Anita's beliefs about the ACA going forward and influenced her sense that public benefits were designed to be withheld. "It's unfair that people with disabilities get denied assistance," she said. "The paperwork is extremely tedious. Not everyone is lucky like us to get free help from a lawyer." Anita also described the experience as a way of being disciplined into understanding the workings of the social safety net.

"It's like [the] government is trying to avoid giving you a payday," she said skeptically, "with the paperwork, interviews, waiting, and everything, they prolong it as long as possible to prevent you from getting assistance. It took my dad a whole year to get disability benefits. That was a whole year without income for him."

In the years following the stroke, Anita's father improved. Eventually he could walk with a cane and speak pretty clearly. He even remarried. His disability check, combined with his spouse's income, brought the family more financial stability.

Anita impressively managed to maintain excellent grades in these difficult years. Several universities admitted her on full scholarship, and she ended up selecting a Chicago-area institution. When Anita and I met in 2013 at a Logan Square coffee shop, she was just finishing her second year of college, traveling back to Detroit to look after her father as often as possible. She was uninsured, and Medicaid expansion had just started in Cook County.

The memory of managing her father's ordeal weighed heavily on her perception of the health care system in general. "I try not to get sick," Anita said, "and if I get really sick, I take aspirin or try to sleep it off. I won't go to the doctor because I know they'll charge a lot of money." That second part had come from a hard lesson freshman year.

Anita came down with a bad fever and visited her university's clinic. She noted, "I was so sick I didn't even think about the cost." But after seeing the doctor and getting prescribed antibiotics, she'd never *forget* the cost. She received a bill for $500. "It took me five months to pay that off . . . I had a fever and was just puking constantly. I wasn't expecting to pay $500." Her subsequent avoidance of health care was a rational response to her past experiences.

When I asked about the ACA, Anita told me, "I'm not really sure it will be that beneficial. I think it will be useful for people who have money to buy health insurance, but not for people with less money." Again, I heard another young uninsured Latino suggest a health care overhaul meant to help them was *not for them.*

"Why?" I asked.

"The way the health care system in America is set up, it kind of pushes people away from going to doctors because they worry too much about the cost instead of their health," Anita responded. "That's why I don't bother going to the doctor anymore. Back in Detroit, I know families that live paycheck to paycheck, and when I saw a chart for prices of insurance with Obamacare, the cheapest I saw was $60 a month. A lot of people still wouldn't want to pay that. If they can barely pay their rent, how can they pay that for insurance?"

Anita was unaware that she was eligible for Medicaid, and she believed that the marketplace was her only option for acquiring health insurance. She spent 2013 and most of 2014 uninsured.

* * *

Sometime later, Anita was chewing on popcorn when she felt—and heard—something break.

"I cracked my tooth," she told me, "and every time I drink something it hurts."

Anita searched the internet for a dental insurance plan, but the very cheapest she could find was $400 a month. She thought she was screwed, until she was complaining to her college roommate, who mentioned casually, "Oh, I applied for Medicaid, you should get on it."

"But I need to go to the dentist."

"That's OK," her roommate said. "They should be able to help you with that, too."

Anita's roommate sat with her at a computer, directing her to Illinois's online Medicaid application website, and guided her through the application process Alan described earlier.

"What made you believe your roommate's advice?"

"He was just really insistent," Anita said. "He's also from Texas. He came from a very similar background as me, and he said he's had a great experience with it, so I figured why not? My tooth hurt really bad."

This simple interaction shows how a health crisis and a helpful member of her college network combined to steer Anita toward Medicaid. Importantly, Anita's beliefs about the health care safety net did not change—it was a change in her circumstances that led her to seek out the safety net as a last resort.

Two weeks after applying, Anita received a phone call verifying the information she provided in her Medicaid application. She recalled the process being easy. "They saw I had work study and a Pell grant, which meant I have maximum need, so they approved me right away and said I'd receive a card in the mail in 14 days."

The problem was that wait. Anita was in enormous pain, and it felt too urgent to wait for the medical card to arrive and then start the arduous process of finding a Chicago-area dentist. So, "I called my dad in Texas and he found a dentist who could give me a filling for $50. It was with silver instead of white fillings, but my tooth was killing me so much I didn't care." Her Medicaid card hadn't even arrived by the time Anita, fresh off a bus to Texas, had gotten her $50 silver filling to replace the one she broke. With her father's help, her tooth pain was gone.

Despite enrolling in Medicaid, Anita never used it. Even when she needed immunizations to get a job at a day-care center, she refrained from visiting a doctor's office and opted instead to get the shots at a university health center for $25. Anita still perceived the health care safety net as a resource only for true desperation. Her roommate may have helped her acquire health insurance, but it was not quite enough to change her perceptions about what it did and who it was for.

College Organizations

One of the biggest reasons Antonio Cerda, a 25-year-old Latino, became a music teacher was to see the joy people express when they've discovered their voice. "It's such a powerful way to release pent-up energy"—Antonio smiled—"and a lot of these kids need it."

In his Philadelphia youth and now in Chicago's predominantly Latino Little Village neighborhood, Antonio had seen and experienced deep poverty. He cited his family's roughest period, after his mother passed away in a car accident. His father had to work overtime, and Antonio took on multiple jobs to help support the family. The pressure to provide income and care for his younger siblings was already overwhelming when, at age 19, Antonio was confronted about his sexual orientation.

A gay man, Antonio told me, "My family knew for a long time before that," but "they must have told my father because one day he confronted me." Antonio recalled his father asking directly, "Are you gay? I heard you talking on the phone with one of your friends."

"Oh yeah? Was it good and juicy?" Antonio retorted, and his father stormed out in anger. Eventually, Antonio's extended family helped broker a "don't ask, don't tell" peace, in which his father wouldn't ask any more questions and Antonio would never talk about his sexuality at home.

For the next several years, Antonio stayed in Philadelphia, working as a music instructor to support his family and going to college for a BA in the arts. Eventually, Antonio felt he had to get out. "I had been spending all this time taking care of everyone around me, and I decided to just start taking care of myself." He saw that living in the Philadelphia area offered no real opportunities for upward mobility. If he really did want to fulfill his dream, to become a choir teacher and train college students, he needed a master's degree. After finding a job as an assistant choir director at a Chicago-area university, he moved to Chicago. The job paid enough to help him share the rent on a three-bedroom with roommates, but it did not provide health insurance.

We met in July 2013, when Antonio was about three months into his time in Chicago. A few months later, Antonio applied for and was accepted to a master's degree program in music education at an Alabama university with a prestigious music education program. It was a pipeline to the career he dreamed about, but moving to Alabama would mean living with only a bare-bones health care safety net. Unlike Illinois, Alabama did not participate in the ACA's Medicaid expansion, which meant that only children, adults with dependent children, the disabled, and pregnant women could qualify. Because the state was concurrently cutting its Medicaid budget by 5% to 10% each year, clinics for the poor had reduced hours and cut staff, which increased waiting times for patients.[3] One Alabama health care advocate I interviewed described their state's health care infrastructure as "unconscionable."

* * *

"Welcome to backwards Alabama!" Antonio greeted me on the campus of his university. We hadn't spoken in about a year, and we had lots of catching up to do. It was the fall of 2014, still hot and humid in Alabama, enough to spur us to make our campus tour short and retire to a restaurant out of the sun. He talked about how he'd found a job at a Target to make ends meet, although that meant getting a car. "Everything is so spread out here," Antonio explained with annoyance. He added, "Every neighborhood seems to have a Target and a gas station and that's it." Antonio lived in a modest two-bedroom apartment with a roommate who also was a graduate student.

Antonio had already built strong ties with the local Latino community. He made friends through church and in the university's gospel choir, which competed in statewide competitions. Singing, itself, was a source of peace and calm for him in this new environment. "When I'm at practice sometimes, I just let it all out," Antonio said and laughed. "The director has to tell me to calm down sometimes."

I ordered another round of coffee and turned our conversation to the topic of health insurance in Alabama. "Where have you gone for health insurance out here?" I asked.

"I use the college health center for things, but it was annoying that they didn't tell the prices of everything."

"Oh yeah, were you stuck with a big medical bill?"

"Thankfully, no. I did try to look into getting on Medicaid out here, but they said I wasn't eligible. Then, I tried looking into Obamacare and then they told me I earned too *little*. Can you believe that?"

The notion of "earning too little" to qualify for assistance from the ACA was quite common in Alabama. Doris Chandler, a health navigator at a local nonprofit explained the situation to me. "Alabama is not a Medicaid expansion state," she started, "so single, low-income individuals like Antonio are not eligible for Medicaid . . . the only assistance the ACA can provide people are the subsidies for the purchase of private insurance."

"Can Antonio get those subsidies?" I asked.

"In theory, yes. In reality, no." Doris was forthright. "To receive a subsidy for private insurance, you still have to pay a portion of the monthly premium. Right now, the cheapest plan available through the Federal exchange in Alabama is $168 per month, and that's after the subsidy. People can't afford that $168 per month. That's how you end up with individuals who can't get assistance. They are ineligible for Medicaid and earn too little to be able to take advantage of the subsidies."

As Doris described, it wasn't that Antonio earned too little to get insurance on the federal exchange. He just did not earn enough to realistically afford even the discounted monthly premium.

Antonio confirmed that his budget was stretched to its limit: "I've already cut back on cable television, I try to spend around $80 every two weeks on groceries, $350 a month for rent, about $100 a month for gas. I just couldn't afford [health insurance], but thankfully I have this thing that helps me get my medications?"

He hadn't mentioned medications in the past, so I asked, "What are you taking medications for?"

Antonio nervously sipped his coffee.

"My partner got HIV, and he told me I should go and get tested." Antonio paused. "So, I went to the health center on campus to get tested. A few weeks later, I got a call from the county health department telling me I was HIV-positive."

* * *

We sat at that coffee shop for hours. Antonio had only disclosed his HIV status to two of his closest friends. None of his family knew yet as he shared his story with me.

"When the county health department told me [I was HIV-positive], they didn't offer any treatment or referrals on where I can go for help. My partner at the time went to [another city] to see a doctor. This is a small town, and he didn't want anybody learning about his status. It was my friend from the university who took me to a social worker at a local health clinic. When I met with the social worker, they were like, 'You seem to be taking this really well.'" He continued, "I was like, 'What can you do?' Why am I mad? I know what I did wrong. Whatever."

The friend who referred Antonio to the clinic was a connection from his university choir group. And he probably saved Antonio's life.

In a state with a frayed health care safety net, social networks were critical for getting people access to help. The clinic Antonio visited was the only available care facility specializing in supporting individuals living with HIV and able to provide the privacy necessary to avoid stigma. The clinic was hidden in plain sight, with a generic name and providing a wide array of health services in addition to HIV care. It looked like any other business in the area.

College referral networks for health care may be informal, but they are vital for the uninsured. They get good knowledge into the hands of people who need it, because interpersonal connections build trust. In this case, participating in his school's gospel choir introduced Antonio to a well-informed student and provided the trust necessary for him to not only disclose his HIV status but also to ask for help with finding a place for care in this conservative state.

"I haven't talked to my dad about it because he's ignorant," Antonio said. "He'll blow this way out of proportion. I can't talk to him. I could probably talk to my aunt, but she's a certain kind of religious person, and I don't want to hear that from her. I could probably talk to my sister about it, but I don't want to. I don't see the purpose because we already have cancer that runs through our family, and that's depressing enough, and this disease right here is not as bad as cancer, but my family is kind of dramatic."

Despite progress in HIV treatment, its stigma remains strong throughout the United States as well as within the Latino community.[4] In his new rural Latino community in Alabama, it would be hard to keep his HIV status private but no harder than the stigma that could come with disclosure. Antonio still regularly participated in choir and maintained plenty of friendships; however, he only shared his status with two friends he trusted enough to be vulnerable with.

As we talked through his supports, Antonio shared that the health clinic "offered support groups, but I didn't want to do it." Part of the reason was that, he described, "after you test positive the county asks you to name all your sexual partners and to provide their phone numbers. Supposedly, it's in confidence, but [with] someone who hasn't had many sex partners [you] can connect the dots. When I was first diagnosed, [news of my diagnosis] was going all around. I don't know who it was, but somebody was telling everybody I had HIV. That was not cool. When that happened, I just told everybody, 'No, it's not true.' I was really cool about it."

The unsettling experience of having his HIV status disclosed without his consent led him to deny the truth and reinforced Antonio's emotional isolation. Unwilling to risk spreading HIV any further, Antonio had stopped dating and seeking relationships, too.

"I work through things on my own," Antonio figured. "I can cope with things very well. I'm very reasonable. I can sit down, break things down in my head; it's more like me taking myself away from the world. I kind of lose touch with people after a while to get well with myself a lot. I guess it's a spiritual thing. I sit down and try to understand it. I take it all in."

* * *

Perhaps the most important service the health clinic provided Antonio was enrolling him in the AIDS Drugs Assistance Program (ADAP). Without ADAP, the medications to manage his HIV would cost tens of thousands of dollars.[5] With it, he could get his medications for $15 a month. "It's one pill a day," Antonio said; "it's three pills in one." ADAP helped stabilize Antonio's life, allowing him to continue school and take care of his health. He even got a small promotion at his job in this period.

Months later, however, the state government significantly cut the budgets of both Medicaid and ADAP, decreasing the supply of assistance to uninsured HIV patients like Antonio. Clinics scrambled to help as many people as they could, transferring ADAP recipients to a subsidized health insurance plan through the ACA if they could afford the premiums.

A staffer at Antonio's clinic, Allison Oak, told me, "If [patients] meet the income qualification where we know they're going to get a fairly good subsidy, then we're going to try and get them on the ACA. It's unfortunate, but we're living in a state where there's a huge budget shortfall in Medicaid and ADAP. By getting [HIV patients] who are able to work and squeeze in that monthly premium [into ACA coverage], we can get more people some kind of assistance with the little funding we have. The ACA has helped people get access to HIV medications, but [what we're doing now is] really just shifting the way we are assisting people in response to the budget problems."

Allison helped Antonio apply for and enroll in an ACA-subsidized health insurance plan—for the same $168 premium health navigator

Doris had used as an example when she walked me through the problem of people "making too little" for ACA coverage in Alabama the year before. "I went from paying $15 a month to $168 a month for my medications," Antonio confirmed. "Allison explained it to me that the state budget was cutting lots of money from Medicare, health care, I don't know exactly, I just remember them saying they were cutting back all this funding. It makes no sense to me why the state would do that, so I applied [for the ACA]. What else could I do?"

"Did the switch to the ACA change anything?"

"I have to really budget accordingly. I can only pay certain things at certain times of the month. It affected a lot. I don't like it. The premium is so high, and it's probably only going to keep getting higher, but out here, there aren't really any other options." To pursue his dreams and finish graduate school and take care of his health, this was just what Antonio had to do.

Alabama state government budget cuts to ADAP pushed thousands of individuals like him off drug assistance programs. Antonio was fortunate that his ties to the local HIV clinic helped him switch to a subsidized plan through the ACA and that his recent promotion made his the $168 premium just barely affordable. Without those two pieces coming together, Antonio would have lost access to his HIV medication. I don't know what he would have done then.

* * *

The last time I saw Antonio, he invited me to join him and a dozen of his choir friends. As people milled around and chatted, one of Antonio's friends turned the music off, lifted his arm, and burst out in song.

"I open my heart to the Lord, and I won't turn back!" sang the young man with a slow, passionate, warm voice that echoed beautifully through the apartment. Giving him room to finish the first line, Antonio and the rest of the group joined in, immediately turning the apartment into a calmer, soothing, and meditative space. When they ended the song, the group had a good laugh, turned the music back on, and the party continued as if nothing happened.

This moment captured the strength, warmth, and cohesiveness of the friendship network Antonio gained through his participation at a university organization. This community not only helped Antonio access health insurance; it also provided him spiritual, emotional, and psychological support for processing his HIV diagnosis.[6] Although Antonio kept his deepest troubles to himself, he was never alone. In places like Alabama, where the safety net has unraveled, tight-knit communities like Antonio's become centers of care for many people with nowhere else to turn.

Despite having benefited from the ACA, Antonio remained skeptical of, even disappointed in, the health care safety net. "I read something that said premiums in Alabama were only going to increase," Antonio said. "That's not cool. It's expensive!"

And it was true: when the ACA went into effect in 2013, Alabamians had three providers from which to purchase health insurance with government subsidies through the federal exchange.[7] In 2016, however, two of the three providers stopped selling plans in Alabama, citing the inability to turn a profit. This left only Blue Cross/Blue Shield, a de facto monopoly. In my last correspondence with Antonio, I learned that he received notice that his monthly premium was going up, from $168 per month to $233.

The future was uncertain for Antonio. Graduation was approaching, and he hoped he could find a job directing a choir. Until then, his survival would depend, in part, on his communities of support at the university and health clinic.

The Power and Limitations of College Referral Networks

The colleges, universities, or community colleges that young uninsured adults attend can be useful sites for the outreach needed to boost health insurance enrollment. As we saw in my respondents' stories, interventions as simple as disseminating flyers or sharing information with student organizations can make a huge difference for an uninsured student in need. Nevertheless, enrollment information isn't enough to increase insurance utilization, as we saw with Anita, who got Medicaid with her roommate's help but got medical care through her father's network in another state.

From 2000 to 2015, the percentage of Latinos among US college students rose from 5% to 14%.[8] More and more institutions of higher education are earning the title of "Hispanic-Serving Institution," or HIS, a title that renders institutions eligible for various Federal grants alongside historically black colleges and universities (known as HBCUs). With these rising numbers and recognition, Latino students on university and community college campuses deserve advocates' attention: the stories from this chapter reveal the power of extending community-based health insurance outreach strategies to college campus settings for all students but Latinos in particular.

In California, the state university system implemented what was called the "health insurance education project."[9] This program trained student educators about the details of the ACA and placed them on the Cal State system's 15 largest campuses. Student educators gave classroom presentations, sent over a million emails, and hosted enrollment events. At the end of their yearlong outreach effort, the percentage of uninsured students had dropped considerably, from 25% to 10%. Many students enrolled in Medicaid, others simply learned more and acquired health insurance through their families, ACA exchanges, or some other means. We can only assume that the information shared through student-educator events traveled more widely among campus networks as attendees passed it along to other campus connections.

Indeed, in my study, the most powerful campus referral for insurance enrollment seemed to be the mundane word-of-mouth referrals that came from classmates, especially when an individual was enduring a health crisis. Young Latinos may remain less likely to seek insurance when healthy, but their existing connections with classmates, instructors, or staff members can become lifelines in times of crisis, helping Latinos overcome their wariness toward the safety net. The stories from this book show that negative past experiences need not permanently dissuade Latinos from the prospects of acquiring health insurance through the state. With the right information broker or advocate, even the most ardent avoiders of the health care safety net may eventually enroll.

Conclusion

In 2021, health navigators hit the streets again, this time to share information about COVID-19 and vaccination in Latino communities, where Chicago's highest infection and death rates have concentrated. "The unique part of it is that it's peer-to-peer," said Lilian Jimenez, associate director of Welcoming Centers for Refugee and Immigrant Services. "Our health navigators are going out into the community and sharing this information. People are not afraid to ask [questions] because these are community members, and they have, you know, *confianza*."[1]

As I write, in early spring 2021, it is still too early to measure the magnitude of the pandemic's effect in many realms, including on health insurance coverage. We do know that outreach campaigns in Latino and African American communities have been essential in fighting misinformation about COVID-19 and vaccination.[2] According to a survey conducted in late 2020, only 24% of black respondents and 34% of Latino respondents planned to get vaccinated against the new virus compared to 54% of whites.[3] To combat the skepticism and mistrust of Latinos toward the COVID-19 vaccines, health care navigators will need more resources. Currently, they are woefully underfunded. For example, the CARES Act of 2020 provided just $3.2 million for health navigators in Latino communities, barely enough to hire 395 navigators to serve a Chicago Latino population of 1.4 million. Each knot in the US safety net is important, and each one is stressed to its limit.

Moreover, funding is not enough. As the stories shared in this book indicate, even if the United States moved to a universal health insurance system, policymakers cannot assume Latinos would automatically enroll. Past experiences with racialized treatment, stigma, poor health outcomes, unexpected premium hikes, complex systems, dismissive bureaucrats, and state agencies of all kinds have bred the tremendous distrust and uncertainty Latinos feel toward the state. Addressing the legacies of state neglect and violence will require a robust system of community-based organizations, on-the-ground outreach strategies, and networks of trust—as well as state follow-through.

This book shows that an intersectional framework must scaffold our efforts to understand uninsured Latinos' health decisions through scholarly research and to affect them through outreach efforts. The social forces revealed by my participants and informing their choices when it comes to accessing insurance included not only those past interactions with state bureaucracies and bad experiences at county emergency rooms but also criminalized informal health care economies, family obligations, job market constraints, and college referral networks. These structures interact in unique ways, raising the importance of identifying connections between these structures rather than placing them in an explanatory hierarchy and address them one by one.

To date, research on Latinos' access to the health care safety net has largely been grounded in the plight of the undocumented and fear of deportation. Certainly, this is a crucial concern, but immigration is only one of many possible structures that Latinos must navigate to seek health insurance and care in the United States. An intersectional approach allows for a more complete description of these social structures and how they produce multiple pathways into and out of health insurance enrollment. This can help researchers better incorporate understudied structures such as gender, sexuality, or the criminal justice system, not as additional variables but as forces operating in tandem with structures of the family, bureaucracy, and labor market to produce program participation. The intersectional framework is also helpful because it operates explicitly from the standpoint of wanting to transform or dismantle oppressive social structures. This work will not be completed by policymakers tweaking the status quo; thus, the audiences for this intersectional work include organizers, activists, and uninsured Latinos themselves.

Throughout my three years of research for this book, I have fomented some ideas I believe are worth pursuing as part of long-term efforts aimed at transforming social structures, particularly the informal health economy, health bureaucracies, patriarchal families, and higher education. Intersectional approaches, by revealing interlocking social structures, also identify multiple entry points for intervention. As the 2020 protest movements throughout the United States have revealed, movements for large-scale structural change never fully fade. Hopefully, either in my lifetime or the lifetime of the next generation, another massive expansion of health insurance to the uninsured will occur. I hope this book will better prepare us to take advantage of the moments when opportunities arise and circumstances shift, as they always do.

Decriminalizing Informal Health Care Economies

Nick and Lynnette's stories in chapter 2 gave us a glimpse into the massive injustices produced by a country with huge police forces and tiny social work communities. For uninsured people, being put in a position of choosing between economic and physical well-being is a lose–lose scenario that all but inevitably involves criminalization of one form or another. With the exception of private entities profiting from the prison industrial complex, most of society has little to gain from putting citizens in perpetually vulnerable positions.

A first step toward transforming this vicious intersectional structure can begin with decriminalizing informal health care economies in tandem with an expansion of health insurance and health care provision in low-income communities. This would mean tamping down enforcement when it comes to things like the purchase of prescription medications, freeing up money from police department budgets (which, on average, constitute 40% of a given city's total annual expenditures) that could be leveraged to ramp up insurance enrollment efforts.[4] Rather than being arrested and gaining the stigma and roadblocks that come with interactions with the criminal justice system, a violation could trigger a connection with a health insurance navigator and benefits that would obviate the need to buy prescription medications through illicit networks. It would erode some of the motivation to sell prescriptions, too, as we saw people like Lynette get into the market in order to eke out enough money for her own health and survival needs.

Equally important, we need to expand efforts to help individuals expunge their criminal records. Not only do many states force ex-offenders to wait until several years after release before they are eligible for expungement, but they also make the process so complex that, without legal help, few of those eligible can actually get their records expunged. Ex-offenders struggling to get jobs and housing but stymied by their records are trapped in a cycle of poverty and crisis that often results in individuals reentering the informal economy or reentering prison. This is also a privatization issue: researchers have shown that, in the digital age, private companies are the compilers of individual criminal record data, profiting from their role by selling criminal background check services to landlords and employers, selling access to mugshot archives, and even charging individuals to have their own mugshots hidden from internet browsers. Private companies are profiting from people with criminal backgrounds, and they cannot be held accountable when they make mistakes that cost people much-needed opportunities.[5]

From Health Bureaucracies to Health Care Organizing

Many of us associate the term *bureaucracy* with words like *cold*, *red tape*, *gatekeeping*, or *indifference*. If we start with an understanding that health insurance bureaucracies have been (and continue to be) hostile, untrustworthy, or abusive toward many uninsured Latinos, it becomes essential to fundamentally transform how we think of and conduct health care service outreach and delivery.[6]

One way to fundamentally transform this structure is to move away from bureaucracies and approach Latino health insurance outreach as community organizing. As the stories in this book revealed, information about a new government program is not enough to persuade individuals with negative past experiences into enrolling. By explicitly including organizing dynamics in outreach campaigns, organizers can do the extra work of providing uninsured Latinos with the intelligence for navigating complex paperwork, as well as empower them by showing they are worthy of high-quality government health care.

Salvador Cerna was the supervisor of the Affordable Care Act (ACA) outreach efforts for the Chicagoland area from 2013 to 2015. He told me, "My background is in community organizing, so I figured, you know what? I'm going to run this as a political campaign and bring everybody together." Sal believed existing networks of community organizations operated on the basis of trust—not trust of government but trust in community organizers who live and work in the places where they are helping people navigate and participate in government. As Sal put it, the everyday uninsured Latino in Chicago "won't know Get Covered Illinois, but they'll know El Hogar Del Nino, they'll know El Valor, they'll know Alivio Medical Center, they'll know Pilsen Wellness Center. And so that trust already that's been there for years, and the fact that they've interacted with some of them directly or indirectly with those organizations, that's what opened up the doors." Sal's vision created a useful shift in Chicago's approach to health care outreach in Latino communities, in which outreach workers approached their roles as patient advocates and community organizers rather than gatekeeping health care bureaucrats.[7]

Many of the positive interactions between health navigators and uninsured Latinos in this study came as a result of Sal's vision. The navigator who approached Lynette in chapter 1, for instance, came up to her at a youth league basketball game at a Boys & Girls Club gym, speaking to her as a fellow community member in a shared community space. The Illinois Department of Health and Human Services deemed its navigator program a success when the state far exceeded its enrollment projections during the first year of the ACA in 2013. Illinois officials projected 241,500 new Medicaid recipients would sign up,[8] but at least 430,000 people enrolled that year. The success of private insurance enrollment through the ACA marketplace was more modest, yet it accounted for another 217,492 people becoming insured in fiscal year 2013.[9]

Some of the most effective stories of outreach in this study came from health navigators who listened to, validated, and helped uninsured Latinos navigate barriers to health insurance. This work went beyond disseminating information. It involved outreach workers taking an active role in helping uninsured clients evade pitfalls and extract benefits from a social safety net designed to discipline them into self-reliance.[10] This is intersectionality in action.

Another promising aspect of piggybacking health insurance outreach onto community organizing is the potential to mobilize Medicaid recipients into a political constituency. This has already occurred among elderly people, who have mobilized as Medicare recipients. Currently, organizations like the American Association of Retired Persons advocate fiercely to protect and expand Medicare benefits. Conceptualizing health insurance outreach as an intersectional community organizing campaign allows one to imagine and aspire for a similar constituency for uninsured people of color. The United States saw snippets of such a constituency arise as Republican repeal efforts nearly ended the ACA in July 2017. Demonstrations to save the ACA arose in cities throughout the country.[11]

Campaigns also center efforts to empower communities rather than restore or shore up state legitimacy; they are inherently about change and who has the power to make change.[12] This is critical, because history shows that the policymakers and the American Medical Association have consistently defended the status quo and derailed efforts to implement universal health insurance. For the foreseeable future, universal health coverage appears untenable.[13] Rather than waiting for policy to change from the top down, structuring Latino health insurance outreach through grassroots community organizing campaigns may prove more useful in meeting communities' immediate needs.

For scholars, this presents an interesting extension of our research on Latino political leadership. This isn't conventional political leadership, but when we take seriously the notion of Latino health care organizing, then organizers like Sal stand out as changemakers in their communities. Nonelectoral forms of Latino leadership have been overlooked, yet they are key in Latinos' relationships with government.

The biggest challenge to the campaign approach is finding the funds to keep health campaigns going in the long term. Most political campaigns are pop-up affairs, lasting months or, at the most, years. Sal Cerna's outreach campaign was seen as a huge success, but the election of Republican governor Bruce Rauner resulted in drastic cuts to ACA outreach across Illinois, and the bulk of Cerna's campaign staff were laid off.[14] It only took an executive order to pull the plug on this campaign (and lend credence to some Latinos' suspicions that the government didn't actually want to provide the benefits). This cautionary tale suggests that funders in the Latino philanthropy world ought to devote greater attention toward building financial capital to operationalize social and cultural capital in their communities. State governments cannot be counted on to consistently fund such enterprises over time.

Transforming Patriarchal Families

Community-based approaches may also help with tackling some of the deeply gendered and patriarchal family dynamics that prioritize the health and economic well-being of men over women. Perhaps the worst of these dynamics is overt physical violence. Feminist scholarship provides some helpful perspectives that emphasize the need to recognize health insurance enrollment not only for abused women as a tool for physical health but also for economic independence.[15] Lacking health insurance means lacking access, in other words, to both health and autonomy. We must target and transform the social conditions rendering so many women physically and economically vulnerable to abuse.

Camila's and Renee's stories in chapter 4 are just two data points among what the American Psychological Association estimates are a shocking 38 million women who experience some form of physical abuse each year in the United States.[16] The social isolation that attends physical abuse is difficult to penetrate, but a coordinated community response model pioneered in Duluth, Minnesota, has shown success. This model builds institutional ties among health care and child protection agencies, local businesses, the media, and clergy in order to intervene directly with abusers and deter violence.[17] Proponents also aim to disrupt the economic dependence rendering women vulnerable by building this institutional network of accountability. For example, recall the story in which Camila's sister called the police on their father, Aurelio. Imagine if, in that scenario, her call had also gone out to Aurelio's employer, local media, and the pastor of their church. Such coordination is no guarantee that an abusive situation can be disrupted, but the collective community attention might prevent further incidents by making them visible sources of embarrassment in multiple sites in the abuser's broader community.

A coordinated response also makes more services and social supports readily available to women experiencing domestic violence. Renee's and Camila's stories offered some examples, such as Renee's sister finding a clinic offering 10 free therapy sessions to help her through the trauma of sexual assault. In a community response model, these individual incidences of assistance can be delivered as a sort of menu of options and supports. A modest intervention goes a long way in the lives of women in great need. A more robust intervention could disrupt abuse, empowering victims to make change with community support.

The most direct solution to the problem of economic dependence and abuse is to expand employment opportunities and affordable housing. For example, women's rights advocates have introduced "sectoral employment strategies" in which companies offering good pay and health insurance benefits are signed up to help recruit, train, and hire women coping with violent households.[18] In one instance, Allstate insurance donated $1.2 million to domestic violence advocacy groups for insurance industry job training and job placement services for domestic violence survivors.[19] Expanding affordable housing would supplement the important but overburdened service provided by women's shelters. Recall that Camila and her mother Lucy felt trapped in Aurelio's house—otherwise, they feared they would be homeless. If we want to help women escape violent patriarchy, there have to be more realistic options than waiting for space to open in a shelter (where, often, male and/or adult children cannot be accommodated alongside their mothers) or hoping there's room on a friend's couch (and another after that). A more robust combination of hotel and housing vouchers, public housing, and expanded shelters might provide more women with realistic alternatives. Additionally, investing in support groups in which women might build connections, from friendships to job leads, and learn from one another in inspirational and unexpected ways offers an inexpensive way for communities to facilitate their agency.

Privacy is another important concern for women seeking help to escape or manage domestic and intimate partner violence. Current legislation, for example, HIPAA (Health Insurance Portability and Accountability Act), protects women from having their medical records and health information disclosed, but abusers within a family can intercept communication materials related to their victims' efforts to seek help. Abusers can easily hire private investigators and use readily available technologies to learn about their victim's activities and locations. Thus far, 36 states have implemented programs like address confidentiality, which enables individuals escaping danger to route their first-class mail to a substitute address and thereby decrease their vulnerability.[20] (Illinois is not one of them.) Tighter regulations on private investigators and enforcement of laws around the use of tracking tech are just part of the creative thinking needed to help maintain women's privacy and safety.

Radical scholars urge us to tackle the root problems of abuse and domination, namely, patriarchy and white supremacy. Tackling culture requires going beyond policy prescriptions and transforming broader societal norms through efforts like those to promote social acceptance of more diverse family structures, gender roles, and sex roles.[21] When it comes to more direct interventions, scholars suggest revising the target of those interventions so that it is not about removing victims from their homes and communities but about removing *perpetrators* and providing support including long-term rental and mortgage assistance so that victims can rebuild in their own homes. Others advocate for changing representations of women by holding the media accountable for victim-blaming and privileging male-dominated perspectives and perpetuating demeaning stereotypes related to sex and gender, race, and class. Endeavoring to change societal norms around the meanings of these social categories will not be a quick fix, nor can one approach fix it all or even fix a single domain. (Again, intersectionality!) But women will remain vulnerable until we uproot some of our most entrenched social structures, including family and gender.

The ACA was never designed to end or even adequately deal with patriarchal family dynamics, but these stories all teach us that expanding women's health insurance access can help—and to do so will require concurrent reforms and interventions across multiple realms of society. Take, for example, the government's response to the September 11 terrorist attacks. For better or worse, this violent attack cost the lives of 2,996 people, affected millions, and sparked sweeping reforms that established the Department of Homeland Security and coordination centers, bringing together information across multiple law enforcement, immigration, and intelligence agencies in order to hasten detection of potential problems and state responses.[22] According to the American Psychological Association, millions of women experience domestic violence every year.[23] This far exceeds the number of citizens afflicted by international terrorism each year, indicating that a coordinated institutional response to the gendered patriarchal oppression would be a wise investment. The problem of domestic violence is far too large and complex for health insurance reform to tackle, yet applying intersectional thinking in this area provides a useful lens as we consider transforming other daunting and interlocking social structures.

Higher Education, Labor Markets, and Health Insurance

Since nearly half of the US insured population receives their health insurance through an employer, access to affordable higher education and the credentials that grant access to individuals seeking such "good jobs" will be another critical expansion effort if we hope to get everyone insured.[24] Recent research, however, indicates that over the past 20 years, the percentage of employers providing health insurance has declined by 15%. Competition for jobs with insurance is only getting stiffer.

An intersectional approach would suggest that bolstering labor unions might help mitigate the decline in employer-provided health insurance. This will be tough for several reasons, including political rhetoric and corporate wrangling to stifle unions and their bargaining power, and the overall decline of union membership in the United States (both a cause and a consequence of the decline in union power). But when 95% of union members receive health insurance through their union-negotiated contracts, it's a fight worth having.[25] In chapter 5, health insurance benefits are one of the most common benefits that unions negotiate for on behalf of their members. Raymundo and Oliver, in chapter 4, exemplify the benefits of union membership for health insurance access, as they were both able to acquire health insurance through contracts negotiated through their respective teachers' and plumbers' unions.

Scholars and organizers could also push to improve the relationship between higher education and labor unions. While this will be more challenging at wealthy private universities, public universities have shown stronger support for unions, with many, for instance, permitting their graduate students to unionize. Public universities also offer more degree programs that channel students to unionized occupations, such as teaching and nursing. It is difficult to imagine a reversal in the decline of employer-provided health insurance in the United States without union activity, but it is not difficult to imagine a multitude of ways to rebuild the intersection of higher education and labor in order to support union enrollment.

University settings should also be treated as central sites for health insurance outreach efforts, as we saw in chapter 5 (particularly regarding the increasing numbers of Latinos entering institutions of higher education, which is likely to be dimmed by the COVID-19 pandemic but may rebound as the immediate danger subsides).[26] The stories in that chapter revealed the importance of information sharing in social networks, especially on college campuses, for helping uninsured students enroll in Medicaid. Outreach efforts would, thus, be wise to consider classroom settings, course syllabi, office hours, and university events as places in which to connect with uninsured Latino millennials.

Toward an Intersectional Competency

Scholars, activists, and policymakers have long searched for alternative concepts to describe health care knowledge that go beyond the hyper-individualized, deficit-based, and pathological notions of health literacy. Terms like *cultural competency, structural competency, cultural health capital, policy intelligence,* and *wisdom* have provided excellent asset-based alternatives aimed at instructing doctors, medical staff, and bureaucrats as opposed to just the low-income uninsured.[27] The findings from this book suggest that bringing an intersectional lens to these alternative measures of health care knowledge frameworks would help advance the field.

Adding what I call "intersectional competency" to medical and health care education could advance efforts to improve knowledge dissemination efforts about the health care system to uninsured communities of color. Extending the work of Patricia Hill-Collins, intersectional competency would represent the ability to observe and identify places or situations in which multiple social structures converge to influence an individual's health care–seeking decision-making.[28] An intersectional competency approach would complement existing frameworks, as it would help medical professionals, health care staff, or health care organizers think beyond their dyadic relationship with the client to the structural interventions extending beyond their particular domain of expertise. For example, the structural competency approach in medical education aims to help medical staff make their interactions with patients more humane and help imagine new structural interventions to improve health outcomes. An intersectional competency approach would take this further by helping medical staff imagine and inquire about *intersectional* structural interventions that go beyond the direct application of medicine.

For instance, medical staff with intersectional competency might help or provide connections for uninsured individuals with criminal records to get their records expunged. I am not indicating that medical staff should be experts in *everything* but, rather, that an intersectional lens could help medical staff use their already keen observational powers to recognize and act upon circumstances when a patient clearly needs more than medical assistance. Intersectional competency built across domains could help put reformers in the criminal justice and health care domains in closer conversation, too. If, as Hill-Collins argues, intersectional structures are powerful through their interlocking character, it is only through interlocking forms of resistance that they can be transformed.

An intersectional competency would help practitioners identify the social structures that are too easily rendered invisible through the discipline-specific training and work environments that professionals, organizers, researchers, or activists tend to operate in.[29] By extending policy and scholarly gazes to the institutions and practitioners that interact with the poor, we unseat narratives that suggest personal failings and cultural pathologies are to blame for decision-making processes that aren't easily legible to institutions. Instead, we put the burden on institutions to change in ways that better address their targeted population's needs, help organizations operate more transparently, and make the interventions legible to the people they are supposed to benefit.

ACKNOWLEDGMENTS

This book would not have been possible without the generous support of the Robert Wood Johnson (RWJ) Foundation's Scholars in Health Policy Program at Harvard University. From 2012 to 2014, the RWJ fellowship provided me the time, resources, and intellectual support to start this project as the Affordable Care Act (ACA) went into effect in January 2013. I am especially grateful to Alan Cohen and the national advisory committee at RWJ who selected me for this once-in-a-lifetime postdoctoral fellowship program. At Harvard, I benefited tremendously from the advice and guidance of Jason Beckfield, Michele Lamont, Kathy Swartz, and Bruce Western, as well as my fellow RWJ scholars Joanna Brooks, Michael Geruso, Daniel Gillion, Tiffany Joseph, Daniel Navon, and Sarah Staszak. Colleagues during my time on the faculty at the University of Wisconsin–Madison also provided written feedback on early drafts of chapters, especially Mustafa Emirbayer, Myra Marx Ferree, Chad Goldberg, Sida Liu, Jenna Nobles, Pam Oliver, and Erik Olin Wright.

At the University of Chicago, Lis Clemens, Melissa Gilliam, Kimberly Hoang, Destin Jenkins, John Levi Martin, and Jenny Trinitapoli provided useful tips and suggestions for improving the manuscript. Ariel Azar, Emily Claypool, Hannah MacDougall, Nisarg Mehta, Jeffrey Sachs, Bikki Smith, and Wang Zoe (graduate students in my first medical sociology graduate seminar at the University of Chicago) also read and provided valuable comments on a draft of the manuscript. I am grateful to the Neubauer Family Assistant Professor program at the University of Chicago, which provided me the time and resources to complete fieldwork, as well as organize a book conference to solicit constructive criticism on an early draft. I am especially grateful to Bernice Pescosolido,

Ben Sommers, and Forrest Stuart for participating in the full-day book workshop, in which each commented on and critiqued a very rough first draft of this manuscript.

Ilene Kalish, Victor Rios, Pierrette Hondagneu-Sotelo, and the anonymous reviewers at New York University Press (NYU) provided constructive feedback and enthusiastic support for this book project. Ilene provided great feedback and editing that made this book far better than what I imagined it could be. I am extremely grateful to the anonymous reviewers for suggesting I engage more with intersectional theory. Victor and Pierrette have been nothing but supportive, and I'm grateful that they invest the time to curate the NYU Press Latino sociology series. I am honored to see my book join this amazing catalog.

Jessica Robinson and Christina Cano skillfully copyedited the manuscript, and Grant Fan contributed peerless research, analysis, and writing about ACA outreach efforts. Letta Page provided excellent copyediting at the final stage of revision. Amada Armenta, Jennifer Jones, Gloria Gonzalez-Lopez, John Robinson, Michael Rodriguez-Muniz, and Saher Selod also provided keen suggestions in different iterations of this book. The manuscript also benefited tremendously from speaking engagements and audience responses at Harvard University, the University of Michigan, the University of Wisconsin–Madison, the University of Pennsylvania, Northwestern University, the University of Michigan, the University of Chicago, the Annual Meeting of the RWJ Foundation, and the Annual Meeting of the American Sociological Association.

Finally, without the love, support, encouragement, and time so graciously bestowed by my wife, Kimberly Kay Hoang, and daughter, Evelyn Hoang Vargas, it would have been impossible to put the finishing touches on this manuscript amid a global pandemic. They are my refuge.

METHODOLOGICAL APPENDIX

The research design for this project aimed to go for more depth than breadth. In contrast to the approach of books like *Uninsured* by Susan Sered and Rushika Fernandopulle, who interviewed 120 uninsured people across multiple states at one point in time, I interviewed and observed 40 Chicagoans regularly over a period of three years. This resulted in 170 semistructured interviews and 200 hours of participant observation. My rationale for this approach was simple. Scores of health care researchers have surveyed and interviewed the uninsured at one point in time, but few have interviewed and shadowed people as they lived their daily lives and made health care decisions over three years. Sociology, in particular, has a long tradition of ethnographers providing up-close portraits of the less fortunate. In this tradition, I embedded myself in four neighborhoods to discover firsthand what people thought of the Affordable Care Act (ACA), how they thought of Medicaid, and how they came to either enroll or remain uninsured for the three-year duration of this project. Many researchers often conduct an interview or two with a research subject and call it a day, but I wanted more than that. From my experience having written an ethnographic book on violence in Chicago, I knew that lots of face time with research subjects, and constantly returning to the field was the only way to get people to share the most vulnerable aspects of their lives.

It is important to note that this particular research design is what was ultimately responsible for generating the theory and evidence introduced in this book. Specifically, this book made use of longitudinal inter-situational shadowing.[1] This ethnographic method involved observing what occurs as uninsured individuals move across settings and situations. For example, I spent time with uninsured individuals during their leisure time and mealtimes, accompanied them to doctor's appointments, shadowed them as they searched for information about the ACA on their personal computers, and sat alongside them as they interacted with health navigators.

Employing longitudinal inter-situational shadowing enabled me to bring temporality into a theory of Medicaid enrollment. By following uninsured individuals across places over time, I show that the process whereby the uninsured enroll or forego Medicaid unfolds more like a series of events on a pathway than a decision made in a moment of time. Longitudinal inter-situational shadowing enabled me to identify how the past informed the present and how the present informed uninsured individuals' orientations toward the future. Most important, this methodology enabled me to discover the centrality of the informal economy, bureaucracies, family, and college referral networks for my respondents. To be clear, I did not begin collecting data for this study with the predetermined goal of theorizing intersectionality. Rather, intersectionality is what best characterized the stories and contexts I observed in the field.

The remainder of this appendix provides an in-depth discussion of the fieldwork methodology as well as how I dealt with the major challenges that arose during data collection.

The Fieldwork

From June 2013 to December 2016, I spent summers, spring breaks, winter breaks, and weekends (while I was teaching during the academic year) in Chicago conducting in-depth fieldwork. The timing of the study was ideal as ACA implementation had begun in the summer of 2013. By low-income uninsured, I mean individuals who earned below the federal poverty rate and qualified for Medicaid.

In year one, I recruited participants by fielding a short screener survey at churches, fast-food restaurants, bars, and coffee shops in four Chicago neighborhoods (North Lawndale, Little Village, Humboldt Park, and Logan Square). This study only uses pseudonyms for individual respondents and the health organizations they used to maintain their privacy. I do not use pseudonyms for the neighborhoods in the study. I selected these neighborhoods to attain racial diversity in the sample. Humboldt Park and Little Village were predominantly low-income Latino, North Lawndale was low-income black, and Logan Square was home to low-income whites.[2] I approached individuals as they exited church services, waited in line for coffee at a shop, or sat at a bar. To avoid sampling on the dependent variable, I avoided recruiting participants at hospitals, clinics, or health organizations. The goal of this study was to explore variation in the ways people sought health care and focusing exclusively on health care settings would have generated a unique sample. By recruiting from these other neighborhood sites, I was able to generate a sample of individuals with diverse past experiences.

At field sites, I introduced myself as a professor conducting research on the ACA. Since it was 2013, the ACA was very much in the public eye and on the minds of many. Thus, most people were happy to engage in conversation. After asking if they were interested in participating in a study, I invited them to take a short screener survey to determine whether they were low-income and uninsured. The screener helped identify uninsured individuals between 18 and 35 years old. This sampling technique resulted in a diverse sample of uninsured single adults that varied in terms of race (white, black, Latino), education (high school vs. college educated), and employment status (employed vs. unemployed). See table A.1 for a description of the sample.

Data collection consisted of (1) informal semistructured interviews and (2) ethnographic observation conducted by shadowing respondents as they lived their daily lives. At the outset of this project, interviews produced little depth from respondents who were hesitant to share intimate details about their health or experiences being uninsured. Thus, I refined my approach and started conducting semistructured interviews for which I memorized a short list of questions to ask respondents during casual

TABLE A.1. Sample Characteristics of Study's 40 Participants

Sample Characteristics	Number	Percentage
Race/Ethnicity		
Black	9	22
White	6	15
Latino	25	62
Age		
21–25	18	45
26–30	15	36
31–35	7	18
Gender		
Female	22	55
Male	18	45
Education		
High School or Less	28	70
Some College	3	7
College Degree	9	23

conversation at social outings, restaurants, coffee shops, or walks and drives through the city. These questions included, What are your thoughts about the ACA? Are you planning to enroll? and If so, why or why not? Additional conversation topics included their past experiences receiving medical care, views of government, employment history, and understanding of health insurance. When respondents' answers yielded interesting findings, I, in turn, followed up with additional questions.

I audio recorded all the semistructured interviews with the respondent's consent at various locations such as the respondent's home, coffee shops, libraries, bars, or parks. Most interviews lasted from 30 minutes to three hours. I attempted to compensate respondents $25 for their time after each semistructured interview. Most accepted compensation after the first interview but declined in subsequent interviews. The rapport I established, from taking an interest in respondents' lives over a three-year period, dissuaded respondents from accepting additional financial compensation.

Next, I conducted ethnographic observations by shadowing respondents as they lived their lives. This meant accompanying them as they ran errands, watched TV, and ate meals, as well as when they sought to enroll in Medicaid or sought medical care. For respondents interested in enrolling in Medicaid, I asked and received their permission to shadow and audio record them as they sought information from clinics, nonprofit organizations, or online through their computer. In total, I observed 15 appointments between respondents and health navigators. I audio recorded respondents using my smartphone from the time we left for appointments until the respondent arrived home. This helped capture respondents' thoughts both before and after the appointments. I also carried a notepad to write down observations and conversations at all times.

Most of the time, I traveled with respondents to appointments via public transportation (train or bus) or sat in the passenger seat of their car. When we entered appointments with health navigators, I introduced myself as a researcher and friend of the respondent interested in learning more about the ACA. I subsequently asked for the consent of the outreach worker to record their interaction. Some navigators granted permission to audio record the appointments; others did not. In situations in which recording was not permitted, I took detailed notes on my phone. While observing the interaction between respondents and outreach workers, I stayed out of the conversation completely. On the car ride home from the appointments, I asked respondents follow-up questions about how they interpreted their experience. Finally, I did not observe or audio record respondent interactions with medical staff such as doctors or nurses out of respect for their privacy. Instead, I accompanied respondents to the hospital or clinic and left with them as they returned home.

Analysis

To analyze the 400 hours' worth of audio recordings from interviews and observations, I relied on a combination of transcriptions and audio file coding. The NVivo software program for coding qualitative data allows for the coding of audio files by breaking up a one-hour audio recording into multiple small segments (ranging from seconds to minutes in length). This feature proved especially useful for coding audio-recorded data from shadowing participants because it helped me capture the emotions, tones, and scenery of those moments. To code the semistructured interviews, I relied on a team of undergraduate research assistants to transcribe them and code them using conventional coding techniques in NVivo. This approach of listening to ethnographic observations, reading interview transcripts, and rereading handwritten field notes enabled me to identify themes and patterns in the data.

The data analysis stage of this project began in 2014, or one year into the project. In order to identify themes, additional questions to ask, or additional sites to observe, I regularly went back and forth between data collection and analysis. This approach helped me identify aspects of respondents' stories or experiences that I was taking for granted (such as a respondents' consistent use of emergency rooms for medical care) and enabled me to return to research subjects with questions to clarify puzzling observations or findings.

A Note on Adopting an Intersectional Framework

Efforts to formalize the study's findings into some form of theoretical framework also began in 2014. The theoretical framing for this project evolved constantly as I tried to publish early findings from this study in journal article form. In journal after journal, from the *American Sociological Review* to the *American Journal of Sociology* and elsewhere, my articles based on these data received rejection after rejection. Reviewers liked the ethnographic evidence but not the theoretical framework.

Over and over again, reviewers asked me to put each of the explanatory variables from each respondent's story into an explanatory hierarchy. One reviewer asked me to focus on age, another on race, another on gender. The end result was rejection after rejection.

The manuscript rejections proved useful in several ways, as they forced me to go back into the field and collect data on some of the holes in the early iterations of the theoretical framework. In particular, reviewers were really pushing me to figure out how politics factored into people's health care decision-making. "The ACA is one of the most politicized social policies in U.S. history," one anonymous reviewer exclaimed, "it has to matter somewhere." At the time, however, I was working with a very narrow definition of politics, that is, affiliation with either the Republican or Democratic Party, but after some conversations with colleagues, I was introduced to the political science literature on policy feedback theory, which conceptualizes poor people's politics as lessons learned from interactions with government bureaucracies and social safety net programs.

It wasn't until receiving reviews on the book manuscript from NYU Press that a reviewer suggested an intersectional framework, and after reading the works of Patricia Hill-Collins and Nikki Jones, everything started coming together for this manuscript. As I fleshed out each case in my study, it became clear that the argument could not be made within the traditional 10,000 word-limit format of a traditional research paper. I gave myself the analytical freedom (and word space) to really flesh out the data from beginning to end for each case. After doing so, I used a large sketchbook to draw out (by hand) the timeline of events that altered the trajectories of people's pathways to care. Collins's theoretical framework provided me an alternative language from which to organize my findings. This process led me to discover the sites where social structures converged to influence respondents' health care decision-making.

This challenging but necessary journey of writing and revision was humbling because it taught me that, during my training in ethnography and theory, I was never introduced to intersectional approaches. In fact, none of the theory courses offered at the sociology departments I've been employed incorporated intersectionality. This is a glaring omission that constrains researchers into writing ethnographies that view the social world as variables or rely more on pure description and less on theory building. As sociology continues reflecting on the theoretical traditions introduced by scholars of color that it has ignored, it is my hope that more departments begin to incorporate intersectionality into its theory and ethnographic methods training.

Fieldwork Dilemmas

Two major challenges arose over the course of the fieldwork for this book that deserve recognition and discussion: (1) instances in which research subjects asked for my help and (2) discerning the truth from individuals engaged in deviant or stigmatized behavior.

Months into data collection for this project, instances arose in which research subjects asked for my opinion or advice on whether or not to enroll in a health insurance plan through the ACA. In these circumstances, I answered each time by saying that I was not an expert on the law and didn't want to give them bad or inaccurate advice. This helped dampen any concerns that I was influencing the enrollment outcomes of my research subjects. As the fieldwork went on, however, it became more difficult from a moral standpoint to withhold assistance to some respondents. For example, Nick Rodriguez and Daniela Salazar were experiencing health problems and could have seriously benefited from enrolling in Medicaid and getting access to prescription medications. These instances created a moral dilemma. Do I provide these suffering individuals with the basic information that might acquire access to medications by applying for Medicaid? Or do I withhold support out of a desire to not influence my research subjects' behavior? I chose the former. In three cases (Nick Rodriguez, Daniela Salazar, and Sandra Chicon), I volunteered information about the ACA that could have influenced each of these individuals into applying.

For these cases, I used myself as an additional data point and collected data on their responses to the information I provided. To my surprise, Nick, Daniela, and Sandra each did not act on the information I provided them. Their past experiences with the health care safety net still dissuaded them from applying for or even inquiring about the ACA. Therefore, in my analysis, these instances became more evidence of the power that past experiences with health care bureaucracies had on people's health insurance–seeking behavior.

Assisting respondents only continued to be an issue throughout the project for the case of Nick Rodriguez, which raises the second point of discerning truth from individuals engaged in deviant or duplicitous behavior. As Nick was often in desperate need of money, suffering from asthma, and engaged in exploiting family members, I provided Nick some assistance in the form of small "loans" of $5 or giving him rides to and from the hospital or train station. I knew full well that I was also one of the individuals in his social network that he was exploiting for some kind of resource. Thus, of all the cases, Nick Rodriguez was the only one I regularly provided small bits of assistance, particularly during the stretch in years two and three when he was homeless for short periods and living out of his car.

Knowing that I could not trust Nick on his word, I relied much more heavily on direct observations of his behavior and data triangulation by interviewing and shadowing his family members, as well as viewing his social media accounts. My ethnography of Nick generated a number of sensational stories, but I only regarded his stories as credible when I either directly observed it or was able to triangulate with multiple witnesses that it had, in fact, happened. This was also true with respect to Nick's criminal behavior. To be clear, I never directly observed nor participated in any of Nick's criminal enterprises. Rather, for both Nick and Lynnette, I triangulated their stories with criminal records searches at Cook County jail, which confirmed the offenses they were convicted for as well as the time they served.

I employed a similar approach for respondents caught in the web of domestic violence, sexual assault, or a stigmatized chronic illness like HIV. For each of these respondents, I conducted additional fieldwork with family members or friends to triangulate the accounts of their crises. Unfortunately, in each of these instances, there was little I could do to help other than to provide an empathetic ear to their tribulations. For these reasons, perhaps, the biggest influence I likely had on respondents was their mental health, as I became an outlet for them to talk about vulnerable aspects of their lives that they often hid from best friends or family members. To be a completely dispassionate and objective researcher in this instance would have not just been unethical or rude; it would also have completely prevented respondents from allowing me into their lives.

As a sociologist, I felt like it was my duty to get as accurate a picture of my respondents' lives while minimizing the degree to which I influenced people's behavior. In this section, I hope to have fully disclosed these processes such that readers know more about my role in generating the data for this book.

To be clear, the goal of this research was to gain deeper insight into the process whereby Latinos come to participate (or avoid) the expansion of a major government program (Medicaid) aimed at improving their lives. As an individual who does not identify politically with either the Democratic or Republican Party, I believed that the most important part of this project was to inform current or future efforts to expand social safety net programs. When I started this fieldwork, it seemed as though health care policymakers operated with an "if you build it, they will come" mentality with respect to ACA outreach. To a certain degree, many people did sign up right away, but the numbers show that millions still have not. The COVID-19 pandemic has only exacerbated these concerns and reminded us that government plays an indispensable role in assisting its citizens through crises. Researchers and policymakers could benefit tremendously from more intersectional ethnographies to better understand why some choose to engage with government benefit expansion programs and why some do not. These concerns were my primary motivation for completing this study, and they guided my reaction and responses to the moral dilemmas emerging from the field.

NOTES

INTRODUCTION

1 The ACA's logic follows largely economic principles. Through Medicaid expansion and the online marketplaces, the ACA sought to create a more balanced risk pool for health insurance companies. When only sick people purchase health insurance, health insurance companies lose money. When healthy people purchase health insurance, however, health insurance companies' profit. The ACA depended largely on a disciplinary mechanism (e.g., the individual mandate and financial penalty for being uninsured) to get citizens to comply with the law. The mandate was predicated on the idea that people respond to financial incentives and, thus, will enroll in Medicaid or purchase their own subsidized health insurance rather than pay a hefty penalty. In December 2017, however, the Republican-controlled House and Senate passed a tax reform bill that repealed the ACA's individual mandate, thereby removing the primary mechanism for incentivizing health insurance enrollment. Repealing the individual mandate placed the health care system on a path back toward its stratified pre-ACA configuration, in which health insurance options for the uninsured were tied heavily to employment. Although it is still too early to tell what effects this will have on the health care system, Medicaid expansion has remained largely intact.

2 Artiga, Orgera, and Damico, "Changes in Health Coverage."

3 In 2013 alone, 2 million individuals filed for personal bankruptcy as a result of unpaid medical bills, making health care the number one cause of personal bankruptcies, outpacing both credit card debt and unpaid mortgages; Austin, "Medical Debt."

4 Doty et al., "Latinos Have Made Coverage Gains."

5 Taubmann et al., "Medicaid Increases Emergency-Department Use."

6 Doty et al., "Latinos Have Made Coverage Gains"; Taubmann et al., "Medicaid Increases Emergency-Department Use."

7 To be sure, a move to universal health insurance would certainly help, however, research on countries with universal programs still shows disadvantages and constraints for low-income people and racial minorities. The problem of unclaimed health insurance benefits persists even in systems with universal care. Siddiqi et al., "Racial Disparities."

8 Pedraza, Cruz-Nichols, and Lebron, "Cautious Citizenship"; Vargas, "Immigration Enforcement."

9   Alvira-Hammond and Genentian, "How Hispanic Parents Perceive Their Need."

10 Alvira-Hammond and Gennetian, "How Hispanic Parents Perceive Their Need."

11 Illinois Department of Healthcare and Family Services, "Medical Programs."

12 Henriks et al., "A Tale of Three Cities."

13 Chicago Metropolitan Agency for Planning, "Community Snapshots."

14 Chicago Metropolitan Agency for Planning, "Community Snapshots."

15 US Census Bureau, "American Community Survey"; Dardick and Reyes, "Latinos Have the Highest Rate of COVID-19 Infection in Illionois."

16 Despres et al., "Communication for Awareness."

17 Martin, "Why Many Latinos Are Wary."

18 Although quantitative studies show that Latinos disproportionately utilize emergency room care, often due to a lack of health insurance, little, if any, ethnographic research has shed light on the dynamics of Latino emergency room usage. For some exceptions, see Lara-Millán, "Public Emergency Room Overcrowding"; Seim, "The Ambulance."

19 Political scientists have long studied racialized policy learning processes, particularly the ways in which social policies are explicitly designed to discourage racial minorities from enrolling in public benefit programs. This literature has long shown that racial minorities tend to have the lowest rates of take-up for government programs like temporary assistance for needy families, supplementary security income, and Medicaid. Mettler, "Bringing the State Back"; Michener, *Fragmented Democracy*; Schneider and Ingram, "Social Construction of Target Populations"; Soss, *Unwanted Claims*, paperback ed.; Soss, Fording, and Schram, *Disciplining the Poor*.

20 This book is certainly not the first to apply an intersectional approach to the study of Latino health. Please see the work of Lopez, Vargas, and Juarez, "What's Your 'Street Race'?," LeBrón and Viruell-Fuentes, Racial/Ethnic Discrimination"; Viruell-Fuentes, Miranda, and Abdulrahim, "More than Culture"; and Zambrana and Dill, "Disparities in Latina Health."

21 Hill-Collins, *Intersectionality*.

22 Cobb and Hoang, "Protagonist-Driven Urban Ethnography"; Rios, "Decolonizing the White Space."

23 The literature on intersectionality is vast and diverse. Choo and Marx-Ferree, "Practicing Intersectionality"; Crenshaw, "Mapping the Margins"; Hill-Collins, *Intersectionality as Critical Social Theory*; McCall, "The Complexity of Intersectionality." For this book, I rely heavily on Hill-Collins's most recent revision of the theory and apply it as a heuristic for discovering intersectional structures affecting Latino health insurance enrollment. Hill-Collins's most recent formulation distinguishes the intersectional approach to social structure from approaches concerned with multiple identity categories. This book relies heavily on Hill-Collins's structural approach. Hill-Collins, *Intersectionality as Critical Social Theory*.

24 Hill-Collins, *Intersectionality as Critical Social Theory*, 234. Hill-Collins's notion of conjunctures is heavily informed by Stuart Hall's notion of articulation. Hall, *Selected Political Writings*, 91.

25 Hill-Collins, *Intersectionality as Critical Social Theory*, 235.

26 Hill-Collins, *Intersectionality as Critical Social Theory*, 47.

27 To be clear, existing research has generated valuable knowledge, such as identifying factors like cultural differences, language barriers, employment status, and documentation status as contributing to the large number of uninsured Latinos. Documentation status has been featured prominently in Latino health insurance research, as many uninsured Latinos are undocumented Mexicans who, by law, are excluded from government benefit programs like Medicaid. The growing presence of immigration enforcement in Latino communities has also contributed to exclusion from government programs. Vargas-Bustamante et al., "Understanding Observed and Unobserved Health Care Access"; Hagan et al., "The Effects of Recent Welfare and Immigration Reforms"; Ortega et al., "Health Care Access"; Ortega, Rodriguez, and Vargas-Bustamante, "Policy Dilemmas"; Perez-Escamilla, Garcia, and Song "Health Care Access"; Vargas, "Immigration Enforcement"; Vega, Rodriguez, and Gruskin, "Health Disparities"; Wallace and Villa, "Equitable Health Systems"; Castañeda and Melo, "Health Care Access"; Gutierrez, "The Institutional Determinants of Health Insurance"; Hagan et al., "The Effects of Recent Welfare and Immigration Reforms"; Jones, Cason, and Bond, "Access to Preventive Health Care"; Joseph, "Still Left Out"; Pedraza, Cruz-Nichols, and Lebron, "Cautious Citizenship."

28 Tukufu Zuberi provides an excellent overview of the history of this epistemology and the ways it continues to inhibit research on racial minorities. Policy-oriented research designs treat the social world as if it's composed of various substances to which individuals have more or less exposure. Structural effects are measured like an individual's exposure to a pathogen, and much value is placed on identifying causal effects from such exposures. Causal evidence is increasingly important as foundations and policymakers invest more in ideas or interventions that have "proven" to be effective. Arvidson and Lyon, "Changes in Health Coverage"; Zuberi, *Thicker Than Blood.*

Scholars have critiqued the pathogen-based conceptualization of social structure in public health research, as it obscures the role of power relations, naturalizes the role of institutions in society, and makes large assumptions about how structural effects operate on the ground. Emirbayer, "Manifesto for a Relational Sociology"; Crenshaw, "Mapping the Margins"; Nelson, *Body and Soul.*

29 See Alondra Nelson and Ruha Benjamin for other elaborations of this form of social science around health. Nelson, *Body and Soul*; Benjamin, *People's Science.*

30 Bracho et al., *Recruiting the Heart.*

31 My approach to studying uninsured relations with the state is informed by the work of Cecilia Menjívar. Rather than viewing the state as a large monolithic

force, Menjívar emphasizes the need for researchers to identify the connections between the state and other social structures. In other words, the state works in conjunction with structures such as the economy, gender, and race, and Menjívar argues that scholars can identify state influence through the ways the state operates in relation to other social structures. Menjívar, *Enduring Violence*.

32 Jones, *The Chosen Ones*; Martínez-Schuldt and Martínez, "Sanctuary Policies."
33 Michener, *Fragmented Democracy*.
34 For an exception, see Cortez, "Latinxs in *La Migra*."
35 Flores-González, *Citizens but Not Americans*.
36 Doty et al., "Latinos Have Made Coverage Gains."
37 Armenta, *Protect, Service, and Deport*; Durán, *Gang Life*; García, *Legal Passing*; Rios, *Punished*; Rios, *Human Targets*; Macías-Rojas, *From Deportation to Prison*; Renfigo and Pater, "Close Call."
38 Parker, "Health Literacy."
39 Ralph, "Becoming Aggrieved." Similarly, Forrest Stuart documents how the "cop wisdom" poor residents exhibit in Los Angeles's Skid Row neighborhood to survive constant surveillance from police is an "unmatched level of creativity, ingenuity, and resilience as they navigate tumultuous conditions"; Stuart, *Down, Out, and Under Arrest*, 21. Similarly, Victor Rios's research on Latino youth argues for the need to reframe them as "at-promise youth" instead of the commonly used term "at-risk youth." Rios, *Human Targets*.
40 Shim, "Cultural Health Capital."
41 Carman, "The Accountability Movement"; Hwang and Powell, "The Rationalization of Charity."
42 INCITE!, Incite! Women of Color against Violence, and Incite! Women of Color against Violence Staff, *The Revolution Will Not Be Funded*; Vargas, "Gangstering Grants."

1. HOW THE UNINSURED ARE CRIMINALIZED

1 Rosenthal, "The Soaring Cost of a Simple Breath."
2 For a great full examination of the intersection of health and criminal justice, see Lara-Millan, *Redistributing the Poor*.
3 For Latino experiences with the criminal justice system, see Lopez-Aguado, *Stick Together*; Peguero and Bracy, "School Order, Justice, and Education"; Rios, *Punished*.
4 Pager, "The Mark of a Criminal Record."
5 Brayne, *Predict and Surveil*.
6 Comfort, *Doing Time Together*.
7 Conrad, "Medicalization and Social Control"; Lara-Millan, "Public Emergency Room Overcrowding"; Lara-Millán, *Redistributing the Poor*; Miller, "Devolving the Carceral State"; Miller, *Halfway Home*; Stuart, *Down, Out, and Under Arrest*; Walker, "Race Making in a Penal Institution."

8 Nick's positive experience with medical treatment should not be interpreted as common or representative of the entire Illinois corrections system. In April 2017, the American Civil Liberties Union of Illinois successfully filed a class-action lawsuit against the Illinois Department of Corrections charging that Illinois prisons do not meet constitutional standards. In 2015, an independent panel of experts issued a scathing 405-page report detailing the poor quality of health care for Illinois prison inmates Overall, prisons, in general, are places with severe inadequacies in health care provision. Walsh, "Does Bad Health Care Constitute"; Meisner, "Independent Experts Blast Quality"; Rich, Wakeman, and Dickman, "Medicine and the Epidemic of Incarceration"; Tabachnick, "Obamacare for Ex-Inmates"; Wilper et al., "The Health and Health Care of US Prisoners."

9 Lara-Millán's ethnography of the Los Angeles County Jail found widespread use of prescription medications to help manage inmate populations. Lara-Millán, *Redistributing the Poor.*

10 Pager, "The Mark of a Criminal Record."

11 Pager, "The Mark of a Criminal Record"; Western, *Homeward.*

12 Matt Desmond refers to this kind of phenomenon as "disposable ties," that is, "relations between new acquaintances characterized by accelerated and simulated intimacy, a high amount of physical copresence (time spent together), reciprocal or semireciprocal resource exchange, and a relatively short life span." He describes it as a survival strategy among the poor. Desmond, "Disposable Ties," 1311.

13 Nikki Jones uncovered a similar pattern of men of color redirecting the oppression they've been subjected to onto women of color. Jones, *The Chosen Ones.*

14 Studies show that people with such negative experiences with the criminal justice system are less likely to apply for public benefits, vote, or engage in civic activities. Burch, *Trading Democracy for Justice*; Massoglia and Pridemore, "Incarceration and Health"; Soss, *Unwanted Claimse*, paperback ed.

15 Watkins-Hayes, *The New Welfare Bureaucrats.*

16 For exceptions see, Miller (2021), Raudenbush, "Health Care off the Books"; Western, *Homeward.*

17 Acri, "Pharmaceutical Counterfeiting."

18 Walter, "Officers See More Sick."

19 Patel et al., "Integrating Correction and Community Health Care."

20 Gates, Aritga, and Rudowitz, "Health Coverage and Care."

2. WHO DESERVES HEALTH CARE?

1 Campbell, "Participatory Reactions to Policy Threats"; Levine, *Ain't No Trust*; Mettler and Soss, "The Consequences of Public Policy"; Michener, *Fragmented Democracy*; Soss, *Unwanted Claims*, paperback ed.; Soss, Fording, and Schram, *Disciplining the Poor*; Soss and Weaver, "Police Are Our Government."

2 Soss, *Unwanted Claims.*

3 In her study of Latino millennials, Flores-González found strong evidence of young Latino adults feeling excluded by US society. Like Telles and Ortiz's study of Mexican Americans across generations in the southwest, Flores-González's study of Mexican Americans in Chicago finds a similar sense of alienation and racialized exclusion. This chapter supports the findings from this previous work and extends it to the realm of health insurance access by demonstrating how such forms of exclusion have consequences for the ability to acquire health insurance. Flores, *Citizens but Not Americans*; Telles and Ortiz, *Citizens but Not Americans*.

4 Soss, *Unwanted Claims*, paperback ed.

5 Watkins-Hayes, *The New Welfare Bureaucrats*.

6 Soss, Fording, and Schram (2009)

7 Du Bois, *The Souls of Black Folk*.

8 Carter refers to this as dominant cultural capital. Carter, *Keepin' It Real*.

9 Studies of Latinos in higher education have similarly found interactions with financial aid bureaucracies to be exclusionary. Diaz-Strong et al., "Purged"; Flores, "Forms of Exclusion."

10 Golash-Boza, *Unwanted Claims*.

11 Sonier, Boudreaux, and Blewett, "Medicaid 'Welcome-Mat' Effect."

12 Marrow and Joseph, "Excluded and Frozen Out."

13 Feagin and Bennefield, "Systemic Racism"; Nelson, *Body and Soul*; Washington, *Medical Apartheid*.

14 National Women's Law Center, "Double the Trouble."

15 Fergusson, Horwood, and Ridder, "Abortion in Young Women."

16 Pandey, "55 Million People Have Access."

17 Holliday, "Logan Square, Avondale Rents."

18 Illinois Department of Public Health, "Illinois Hospital Report Card."

19 Bradley and Taylor, *The American Health Care Paradox*.

20 Colorado Department of Health Care Financing, "General Requirements to Qualify"; Centers for Medicare and Medicaid Services, "Managed Care."

21 Kliff, "Want to Reverse Obamacare's Cancellations?"

22 The positive effects of acquiring health insurance on mental health have been documented in other studies. Baicker and Finkelstein, "The Effects of Medicaid Coverage."

23 Leys, "Iowa Medicaid Payment Shortages."

24 Soss, Fording, and Schram (2009).

25 Since the publication of Gans's book, the war on the poor has arguably continued in an evolved manner through trends like increased policing, surveillance, immigration enforcement, and labor market deregulation, to name a few. Gans, *The War against the Poor*.

3. WHY LATINA WOMEN SACRIFICE THEIR COVERAGE

1 Flores-González, *Citizens but Not Americans*; Lopez, Krogstad, and Flores, "Key Facts about Young Latinos."

2 Milkman, "A New Political Generation."

3 Milkman, "A New Political Generation."

4 Scholars have studied similar patriarchal dynamics within Latino families. This chapter builds on and extends this line of research by investigating the consequences of these patriarchal family structures for health insurance access. Flores-González, *Citizens but Not Americans*; Gonzáles-López, *Family Secrets*; Gonzales, *Lives in Limbo*; Hondagneu-Sotelo, *Gendered Transitions*; Smith, *Mexican New York*; Vasquez, *Mexican Americans across Generations*.

5 State of Illinois, "Candidate's Guide."

6 Royner, "Health Care's a Big Issue."

7 Bourgeois, Schulz, and Burgio, "Interventions for Caregivers."

8 Wogan, "Who's an Employee?"

9 In her study of Mexican migration experiences, Hondagenou-Sotelo found that migrants like Renee's father are often burdened with medical debt. Moreover, the masculinized dignity of working through pain and injury may also be factors behind Renee's father's resistance to provide health insurance for her. Hondagneu-Sotelo, *Gendered Transitions*. Also see Walter, Bourgois, and Loinaz, "Masculinity and Undocumented Labor Migration."

10 Similar dynamics have been found in the study of first-generation college students and their immigrant working-class parents. Rondini, "Healing the Hidden Injuries."

11 Rape, Abuse & Incest National Network, "Victims of Sexual Violence Statistics."

12 Granovetter, "The Strength of Weak Ties"; Montgomery, "Job Search and Network Composition."

13 González-López, *Family Secrets*.

14 Illinois Department of Children and Family Services, "Day Care Homes."

15 Illinois Department of Children and Family Services, "Day Care Homes."

16 Savage, "What to Do if You Can't Afford Obamacare."

17 Across the country, the price of premiums in health insurance markets has been steadily increasing in states like Illinois. Policymakers and scholars attribute this to the fact that unhealthy individuals were largely the first to purchase subsidized plans that , in turn, resulted in high usage and submission of large claims. When these circumstances are combined with fewer healthy people signing up and political uncertainty in Washington, D.C., over the long-term stability of the ACA, prices increase. Sonier, Boudreaux, and Blewett, "Medicaid 'Welcome-Mat' Effect." Baker, Bloom, and Davis, "Measuring Economic Policy Uncertainty."

18 For a much deeper interstate analysis of experiences with Medicaid, see Michener, *Fragmented Democracy*.

19 Winston's logic is not entirely incorrect. Through Medicaid expansion and the online marketplaces, the ACA sought to create a more balanced risk pool for health insurance companies. When only sick people purchase health insurance, this creates a problem that economists call adverse selection, which results in higher prices for health care. By mandating that everyone purchase health insurance, the ACA aimed to get more healthy people to purchase health insurance, which, in turn, would help slow the growing cost of health care. The ACA depended largely on a disciplinary mechanism, that is, the threat of a financial penalty for being uninsured to get citizens to comply with the law. When the ACA went into effect in 2014, however, the minimum penalty for an uninsured adult was $95, an amount many felt was too little to incentivize the uninsured into acquiring health insurance. Pear, "Health Care Penalty?".

   In December 2017, however, the Republican-controlled House and Senate passed a tax reform bill that repealed the ACA's mandate, which eradicated the financial penalty. Repealing the financial penalty has placed the health care system on a path back toward its stratified pre-ACA configuration, whereby access to health insurance for the uninsured is tied heavily to employment. Jost, "Examining the House Republican ACA Repeal and Replace Legislation."

20 Soss, Fording, and Schram, *Disciplining the Poor*.

21 Susan Sered describes the pain management strategies in her book *Uninsured in America*.

22 This finding corroborates Jamila Michener's research on the significance of place for understanding Medicaid enrollment and political orientations toward Medicaid. Michener, *Fragmented Democracy*.

23 Bracho et al., *Recruiting the Heart*.

24 Parreñas, *Servants of Globalization*.

25 Ortiz, "Shortage of Caregivers."

26 Berens and Callahan, "In Illinois Group Homes, Adults with Disabilities Suffer."

27 Lorber, *Breaking the Bowls*; Risman, "From Doing to Undoing."

4. THE ROLE GENDER PLAYS IN ACCESS TO HEALTH CARE

1 In her study of patriarchal relationships in Mexican families where incestuous sexual violence exists, Gloria Gonzalez-Lopez describes the role of the conjugal daughter as someone who becomes "like a spouse to one of their parents," usually the father, as part of a larger pattern of emotional abuse and neglect in the family. A "parental child" is the one who "becomes a parent to siblings." González-López, *Family Secrets*.

2 Camila's experience with the police was a best-case scenario. Women who have called Chicago police for assistance with a violent family member have been subjected to being interviewed in front of their abuser, left alone with their abuser after police declined to make an arrest, or had the abuser answer police questions when the victim could not speak English. Jones, "Police Dig Deeper."

3 The lack of institutional support for helping Camila and her family escape Aurelio reflects what feminist state theorists call the "patriarchal state." Like the health care safety net's inability to help temp workers, the welfare state is unequipped to support women dependent on abusers. Some argue that the state's inadequacy is not a coincidence but, rather, a reflection of the state's interest in regulating women's bodies and desires. Mink, *Welfare's End*; Scott, London, and Myers, "Dangerous Dependencies"; Haney, *Offending Women*.

4 Illinois Department of Human Services, "Domestic Violence Agencies by City."

5 This instance, again, shows the importance of Small's notion of organizational embeddedness, as the referral from a friend at the nonprofit is what ultimately sparked the sequence of events that led Camila to Medicaid. Small, *Unanticipated Gains*.

6 It's difficult to pin down exactly why Camila's and Renee's mothers differed in the ways they supported their daughters. The most noticeable difference was where they were born. Renee's mother was born in the same rural Mexican town as her father and was thus raised in a setting in which these patriarchal dynamics were much more pervasive. Camila's mother, in contrast, was born and raised in Chicago, where patriarchal dynamics are certainly present but not in the same form as in rural Mexican towns.

7 González-López refers to such processes as a form of "internalized sexism." González-López, *Family Secrets*.

8 Villa-Torres, Fleming, and Barrington, "Engaging Men as Promotores de Salud."

9 Bracho et al., *Recruiting the Heart*.

5. THE POWER OF SOCIAL NETWORKS TO SECURE INSURANCE

1 Levine and Mulligan, "Mere Mortals."

2 Small, *Unanticipated Gains*.

3 Lyman, "Senate's Proposed Medicaid Cuts."

4 Derose et al., "An Intervention to Reduce HIV-Related Stigma."

5 Nall, Holland, and Cherney, "The Cost of HIV Treatment."

6 This corroborates research findings on the beneficial effects of collective efficacy (or community trust and cohesion) on health outcomes. Browning and Cagney, "Neighborhood Structural Disadvantage."

7 Booker and Kargbo, "Alabama Residents Left with One Insurance Option under ACA."

8 Vargas, "Racial Expropriation in Higher Education."

9 Zelman, "College Campuses Are Fertile Ground."

CONCLUSION

1 Zamudo, "How Promotoras Are Fighting."

2 Chase, "Coronavirus Crippling Chicago's Census Outreach Effort."

3 Neegaard and Fingerhut, "AP-NORC Poll."

4 Badger and Bui, "Cities Grew Safer."

5 Lageson, *Digital Punishment*; Middlemass, *Convicted and Condemned.*

6 Nelson, *Body and Soul.*

7 Bracho et al., *Recruiting the Heart.*

8 Institute for Illinois' Fiscal Sustainability at the Civic Federation, "Illinois Medicaid Enrollment."

9 Institute for Illinois' Fiscal Sustainability at the Civic Federation, "Illinois Medicaid Enrollment."

10 Soss, Fording, and Schram, *Disciplining the Poor.*

11 DeBonis and Wiegel, "Activist Muscle Gives Obamacare a Lift."

12 For an excellent study of how community organizers can still secure resources for their community amidst strong distrust of local government, see Gonzales's *Building a Better Chicago.*

13 Starr, *Social Transformation of American Medicine.*

14 Davey, "Illinois Governor Proposes $6 Billion in Cuts"; Bosman and Davey, "Everything's in Danger."

15 Houston, "How Feminist Theory Became (Criminal) Law"; Renzetti, "On Dancing with a Bear"; Villavon, *Violence against Latina Immigrants.*

16 American Psychological Association, "Intimate Partner Abuse."

17 Pence and McMahon, "Duluth."

18 Correia, "Strategies to Expand Battered Women's Economic Opportunities."

19 Engage for Good, "1 in 4 Women Experience Domestic Violence."

20 National Center for Victims of Crime, "Address Confidentiality Programs."

21 Lorber, *Breaking the Bowls*; Risman, "From Doing to Undoing."

22 Foner, *Wounded City.*

23 American Psychological Association, "Intimate Partner Abuse."

24 Lin, Bondurant, and Messamore, "Union."

25 US Bureau of Labor Statistics, "Union Workers More Likely than Nonunion Workers to Have Healthcare."

26 Zarate and Gallimore, "Gender Differences in Factors Leading to College Enrollment."

27 Metzl and Hansen, "Structural Competency"; Shim, "Cultural Health Capital"; Stuart, *Down, Out, and Under Arrest.*

28 Hill-Collins, *Intersectionality as Critical Social Theory.*

29 Metzl and Hansen, "Structural Competency."

METHODOLOGICAL APPENDIX

1 Trouille and Tavory, "Shadowing."

2 Since the completion of data collection, Logan Square has undergone significant gentrification. Thus, much of the low-income population has likely left by now.

REFERENCES

Acri, Kristina M. L. 2018. "Pharmaceutical Counterfeiting: Endangering Public Health, Society, and the Economy." Vancouver, CA: Fraser Institute. https://www.fraserinstitute.org.

Alvira-Hammond, Marta, and Lisa A Gennetian. 2015. "How Hispanic Parents Perceive Their Need and Eligibility for Public Assistance." National Research Center on Hispanic Children and Families. www.hispanicresearchcenter.org.

American Psychological Association. 2018. "Intimate Partner Abuse and Relationship Violence." https://www.apa.org.

Armenta, Amada. 2017. *Protect, Serve, and Deport: The Rise of Policing as Immigration Enforcement.* Oakland: University of California Press.

Artiga, Samantha, Kendal Orgera, and Anthony Damico. 2020. "Changes in Health Coverage by Race and Ethnicity since the ACA, 2010–2018." Kaiser Family Foundation, March 5. https://www.kff.org.

Arvidson, Malin, and Fergus Lyon. 2014. "Social Impact Measurement and Non-Profit Organisations: Compliance, Resistance, and Promotion." *VOLUNTAS: International Journal of Voluntary and Nonprofit Organizations* 25 (4): 869–86.

Austin, Daniel. 2014. "Medical Debt as a Cause of Consumer Bankruptcy." *Maine Law Review* 67 (1): 1–23.

Baciker, Katherine, and Amy Finklestein. 2011. "The Effects of Medicaid Coverage: Learning from the Oregon Experiment." *New England Journal of Medicine* 365 (8): 683–85.

Badger, Emily, and Quoctrung Bui. 2020. "Cities Grew Safer. Police Budgets Kept Growing." *New York Times*, June 12. https://www.nytimes.com.

Baker, Scott R., Nicholas Bloom, and Steven J. Davis. 2016. "Measuring Economic Policy Uncertainty." *Quarterly Journal of Economics* 131 (4): 1593–636.

Benjamin, Ruha. 2013. *People's Science: Bodies and Rights on the Stem Cell Frontier.* Palo Alto, CA: Stanford University Press.

Berens, Michael J., and Patricia Callahan. 2016. "In Illinois Group Homes, Adults with Disabilities Suffer." *Chicago Tribune*, November 17. https://www.chicagotribune.com.

Booker, Christopher, and Connie Kargbo. 2017. "Alabama Residents Left with One Insurance Option under ACA." PBS Newshour, June 17. NPR. Transcript. https://pbs.org.

Bosman, Julie, and Monica Davey. 2017. "Everything's in Danger: Illinois Approaches 3rd Year without Budget." *New York Times*, June 29. https://www.nytimes.com.

Bourgeois, Michelle S., Richard Schulz, and Louis Burgio. 1996. "Interventions for Caregivers of Patients with Alzheimer's Disease: A Review and Analysis of Content, Process, and Outcomes." *The International Journal of Aging and Human Development* 43 (1): 35–92.

Bracho, America, Ginger Lee, Gloria Giarldo, Rosa Maria De Prado, and the Latino Health Access Collective. 2016. *Recruiting the Heart, Training the Brain: The Work of Latino Health Access*. Berkeley, CA: Hesperian Health Guides.

Bradley, Elizabeth H., and Lauren A. Taylor. 2013. *The American Health Care Paradox: Why Spending More Is Getting Us Less*. New York: PublicAffairs.

Brayne, Sarah. 2020. *Predict and Surveil: Data, Discretion, and the Future of Policing*. New York: Oxford University Press.

Browning, Christopher R., and Kathleen A. Cagney. 2002. "Neighborhood Structural Disadvantage, Collective Efficacy, and Self-Rated Physical Health in an Urban Setting." *Journal of Health and Social Behavior* 43 (4): 383–99.

Burch, Traci. 2013. *Trading Democracy for Justice: Criminal Convictions and the Decline of Neighborhood Political Participation*. Chicago: University of Chicago Press.

Campbell, Andrea Louise. 2003. "Participatory Reactions to Policy Threats: Senior Citizens and the Defense of Social Security and Medicare." *Political Behavior* 25 (1): 29–49.

Carman, Joanne G. 2010. "The Accountability Movement: What's Wrong with This Theory of Change?" *Nonprofit and Voluntary Sector Quarterly* 39 (2): 256–74.

Carter, Prudence L. 2005. *Keepin' It Real: School Success Beyond Black and White*. New York: Oxford University Press.

Castañeda, Heide, and Milena Andrea Melo. 2014. "Health Care Access for Latino Mixed-Status Families: Barriers, Strategies, and Implications for Reform." *American Behavioral Scientist* 58 (14): 1891–909.

Centers for Medicare and Medicaid Services. 2018. "Managed Care." Baltimore: Centers for Medicare & Medicaid Services. https://www.medicaid.gov.

Chase, Brett. 2020. "Coronavirus Crippling Chicago's Census Outreach Effort." Better Government Association, March 23. https://www.bettergov.org.

Chicago Metropolitan Agency for Planning. 2020. "Community Snapshots." Chicago: Chicago Metropolitan Agency for Planning. https://www.cmap.illinois.gov.

Choo, Hae Yeon, and Myra Marx Ferree. 2010. "Practicing Intersectionality in Sociological Research: A Critical Analysis of Inclusions, Interactions, and Institutions in the Study of Inequalities." *Sociological Theory* 28 (2): 129–49.

Cobb, Jessica Shannon, and Kimberly Kay Hoang. 2015. "Protagonist-Driven Urban Ethnography." *City & Community* 14(4): 348–51.

Colorado Department of Health Care Policy and Financing. 2016. "General Requirements to Qualify for Medical Assistance." Denver: Colorado Department of Health Care Policy and Financing. https://www.colorado.gov.

Comfort, Megan. 2009. *Doing Time Together: Love and Family in the Shadow of the Prison*. Chicago: University of Chicago Press.

Conrad, Peter. 1992. "Medicalization and Social Control." *Annual Review of Sociology* 18 (1): 209–32.

Correia, Amy. 2000. "Strategies to Expand Battered Women's Economic Opportunities." Publication #9. Harrisburg, PA: National Resource Center on Domestic Violence. http://www.vawnet.org.

Cortez, David. 2020. "Latinxs in *La Migra*: Why They Join and Why It Matters." *Political Research Quarterly*. Published ahead of print, June 25. doi:10.1177/1065912920933674

Crenshaw, Kimberlé. 1991. "Mapping the Margins: Intersectionality, Identity Politics, and Violence Against Women of Color." *Stanford Law Review* 43 (6): 1241–99.

Dardick, Hall, and Cecilia Reyes. 2020. "Latinos Have the Highest Rate of COVID-19 Infection in Illinois." *Chicago Tribune*, June 5. http://www.chicagotribune.com

Davey, Monica. 2015. "Illinois Governor Proposes $6 Billion in Cuts and Reducing Pension Benefits." *New York Times*, February 19. https://www.nytimes.com.

DeBonis, Mike, and David Wiegel. 2017. "Activist Muscle Gives Obamacare a Lift." *Washington Post*, February 25. https://www.washingtonpost.com.

Derose, Kathryn Pitkin, Laura M. Bogart, David E Kanouse, Alexandria Felton, Deborah Owens Collins, Michael A. Mata, Clyde W. Oden, Blanca X. Domínguez, Karen R. Flórez, and Jennifer Hawes-Dawson. 2014. "An Intervention to Reduce HIV-Related Stigma in Partnership with African American and Latino Churches." *AIDS Education and Prevention* 26 (1): 28–42.

Desmond, Matthew. 2012. "Disposable Ties and the Urban Poor." *American Journal of Sociology* 117 (5): 1295–335.

Despres, Cliff, Rosalie Aguilar, Alfred McAlister, and Amelie G Ramirez. 2020. "Communication for Awareness and Action on Inequitable Impacts of COVID-19 on Latinos." *Health Promotion Practice* 21 (6): 859–61.

Diaz-Strong, Daysi, Christina Gómez, Maria E. Luna-Duarte, and Erica R. Meiners. 2011. "Purged: Undocumented Students, Financial Aid Policies, and Access to Higher Education." *Journal of Hispanic Higher Education* 10 (2): 107–19.

Doty, Michelle M., Sophie Beutel, Petra W. Rasmussen, and Sara R. Collins. 2015. "Latinos Have Made Coverage Gains but Millions Are Still Uninsured." *The Commonwealth Fund Blog*, April 27. https://www.commonwealthfund.org.

Du Bois, W. E. B. (1903) 2017. *The Souls of Black Folk*. Scotts Valley, CA: CreateSpace.

Durán, Robert. 2013. *Gang Life in Two Cities: An Insider's Journey*. New York: Columbia University Press.

Emirbayer, Mustafa. 1997. "Manifesto for a Relational Sociology." *American Journal of Sociology* 103 (2): 281–317.

Engage for Good. 2018. "1 in 4 Women Experience Domestic Violence, but Americans Are Less Likely to Discuss the Issue Today than 4 Years Ago." https://engageforgood.com.

Feagin, Joe, and Zinobia Bennefield. 2014. "Systemic Racism and U.S. Health Care." *Social Science & Medicine* 103 (1): 7–14.

Fergusson, D. M., L. John Horwood, and E. M. Ridder. 2006. "Abortion in Young Women and Subsequent Mental Health." *Journal of Child Psychology and Psychiatry* 47 (1): 16–24.

Flores, Andrea. 2016. "Forms of Exclusion: Undocumented Students Navigating Financial Aid and Inclusion in the United States." *American Ethnologist* 43 (3): 540–54.

Flores-González, Nilda. 2017. *Citizens but Not Americans: Race and Belonging among Latino Millennials*. New York: New York University Press.

Foner, Nancy. 2005. *Wounded City: The Social Impact of 9/11 on New York City*. New York: Russell Sage Foundation.

Gans, Herbert J. 1995. *The War against the Poor: The Underclass and Antipoverty Policy*. New York: Basic Books.

García, Angela S. 2019. *Legal Passing: Navigating Undocumented Life and Local Immigration Law*. Berkeley: University of California Press.

Gates, Alexandra, Samantha Artiga, and Robin Rudowitz. 2014. "Health Coverage and Care for the Adult Criminal Justice-Involved Population." The Henry J. Kaiser Family Foundation, September 5. https://www.kff.org.

Golash-Boza, Tanya Maria. 2012. *Immigration Nation: Raids, Detentions, and Deportations in Post-9/11 America*. Boulder, CO: Paradigm Publishers.

Gonzales, Roberto G. 2016. *Lives in Limbo: Undocumented and Coming of Age in America*. Berkeley: University of California Press.

Gonzales, Teresa Irene. 2021. *Building a Better Chicago: Race and Community Resistance to Urban Redevelopment*. New York University Press.

González-López, Gloria. 2015. *Family Secrets: Stories of Incest and Sexual Violence in Mexico*. New York: New York University Press.

Granovetter, Mark S. 1973. "The Strength of Weak Ties." *American Journal of Sociology* 78 (6): 1360–80.

Gutierrez, Carmen M. 2018. "The Institutional Determinants of Health Insurance: Moving Away from Labor Market, Marriage, and Family Attachments under the ACA." *American Sociological Review* 83 (6): 1144–70.

Hagan, Jacqueline, Nestor Rodriguez, Randy Capps, and Nika Kabiri. 2003. "The Effects of Recent Welfare and Immigration Reforms on Immigrants' Access to Health Care." *International Migration Review* 37 (2): 444–63.

Hall, Stuart. 2017. *Selected Political Writings: The Great Moving Right Show and Other Essays*. Durham, NC: Duke University Press.

Haney, Lynne A. 2010. *Offending Women: Power, Punishment, and the Regulation of Desire*. Berkeley: University of California Press.

Henricks, Kasey, Amanda E. Lewis, Iván Arenas, and Deana G. Lewis. 2017. "A Tale of Three Cities: The State of Racial Justice in Chicago." Chicago: University of Illinois at Chicago Institute for Research on Race and Public Policy. https://stateofracialjusticechicago.com/.

Hill-Collins, Patricia. 2019. *Intersectionality as Critical Social Theory*. Durham, NC: Duke University Press.

Holliday, Darryl. 2015. "Logan Square, Avondale Rents Are Through the Roof, Market Analysis Confirms." *DNA Info*, July 2. https://www.dnainfo.com.

Hondagneu-Sotelo, Pierrette. 1994. *Gendered Transitions: Mexican Experiences of Immigration*. Berkeley: University of California Press.

Houston, Claire. 2014. "How Feminist Theory Became (Criminal) Law: Tracing the Path to Mandatory Criminal Intervention in Domestic Violence Cases." *Michigan Journal of Gender & Law* 21 (2): 217–72.

Hwang, Hokyu, and Walter W. Powell. 2009. "The Rationalization of Charity: The Influences of Professionalism in the Nonprofit Sector." *Administrative Science Quarterly* 54 (2): 268–98.

Illinois Department of Children and Family Services. 2017. "Day Care Homes and Group Day Care Homes: Policies, Procedures, and Code Requirements of the Office of the State Fire Marshal." https://www2.illinois.gov

Illinois Department of Healthcare and Family Services. 2016. "Medical Programs." Springfield: Illinois Department of Healthcare and Family Services. https://www.illinois.gov.

Illinois Department of Human Services. 2016. "Domestic Violence Agencies by City." Springfield: Illinois Department of Human Services. http://www.dhs.state.il.us.

Illinois Department of Public Health. 2016. "Illinois Hospital Report Card and Consumer Guide to Health Care." Springfield: Illinois Department of Public Health. http://www.healthcarereportcard.illinois.gov.

Institute for Illinois' Fiscal Sustainability at the Civic Federation. 2014. "Illinois Medicaid Enrollment under Affordable Care Act Exceeds Projections." Chicago: Institute for Illinois' Fiscal Sustainability at the Civic Federation. https://www.civicfed.org.

INCITE!, Incite! Women of Color against Violence, and Incite! Women of Color against Violence Staff. 2007. *The Revolution Will Not Be Funded: Beyond the Nonprofit Industrial Complex*. Boston: South End Press.

Jones, Diana N. 2014. "Police Dig Deeper on Domestic Violence Calls." *Chicago Sun-Times*, October 26. https://chicago.suntimes.com.

Jones, Mary Elaine, Carolyn L. Cason, and Mary Lou Bond. 2002. "Access to Preventive Health Care: Is Method of Payment a Barrier for Immigrant Hispanic Women?" *Women's Health Issues* 12 (3): 129–37.

Jones, Nikki. 2018. *The Chosen Ones: Black Men and the Politics of Redemption*. Berkeley: University of California Press.

Joseph, Tiffany D. 2017. "Still Left Out: Healthcare Stratification under the Affordable Care Act." *Journal of Ethnic and Migration Studies* 43 (12): 2089–107.

Jost, Timothy. 2017. "Examining the House Republican ACA Repeal and Replace Legislation." *Health Affairs Blog*, March 7. https://www.healthaffairs.org.

Kliff, Sarah. 2013. "Want to Reverse Obamacare's Cancellations? Then You're Going to Have to Raise Premiums." *Washington Post*, November 11. https://www.washingtonpost.com.

Lageson, Sarah Esther. 2020. *Digital Punishment: Privacy, Stigma, and the Harms of Data-Driven Criminal Justice*. Oxford, UK: Oxford University Press.

Lara-Millán, Armando. 2014. "Public Emergency Room Overcrowding in the Era of Mass Imprisonment." *American Sociological Review* 79 (5): 866–87.

———. 2021. *Redistributing the Poor: Jails, Hospitals, and the Crisis of Law and Fiscal Austerity*. New York: Oxford University Press.

LeBrón, Alana M. W., and Edna A. Viruell-Fuentes. 2020. "Racial/Ethnic Discrimination, Intersectionality, and Latina/o Health." In *New and Emerging Issues in Latinx Health*, edited by Airín D. Martínez and Scott D. Rhodes, 295–320. New York: Springer Publishing.

Levine, Deborah, and Jessica Mulligan. 2017. "Mere Mortals: Overselling the Young Invincibles." *Journal of Health Politics, Policy and Law* 42 (2): 387–407.

Levine, Judith. 2013. *Ain't No Trust: How Bosses, Boyfriends, and Bureaucrats Fail Low-Income Mothers and Why It Matters*. Berkeley: University of California Press.

Leys, Tony. 2016. "Iowa Medicaid Payment Shortages Are 'Catastrophic,' Private Managers Tell State." *Des Moines Register*, December 21. https://www.desmoinesregister.com.

Lin, Ken-Hou, Samuel Bondurant, and Andrew Messamore. 2018. "Union, Premium Cost, and the Provision of Employment-Based Health Insurance." *Socius* 4: 1–11. https://journals.sagepub.com/doi/pdf/10.1177/2378023118798502.

Lopez, Mark Hugo, Jens Manuel Krogstad, and Antonio Flores. 2018. "Key Facts about Young Latinos, One of the Nation's Fastest-Growing Populations." Pew Research Center, September 13. https://www.pewresearch.org.

López, Nancy, Edward Vargas, Melina Juarez, Lisa Cacari-Stone, and Sonia Bettez. 2018. "What's Your 'Street Race'? Leveraging Multidimensional Measures of Race and Intersectionality for Examining Physical and Mental Health Status Among Latinxs." *Sociology of Race and Ethnicity* 4 (1): 49–66.

Lopez-Aguado, Patrick. 2018. *Stick Together and Come Back Home: Racial Sorting and the Spillover of Carceral Identity*. Berkeley: University of California Press.

Lorber, Judith. 2005. *Breaking the Bowls: Degendering and Feminist Change*. New York: W. W. Norton & Company.

Lyman, Brian. 2017. "Senate's Proposed Medicaid Cuts Worry Alabama Health Care Providers." *Montgomery Advertiser*, June 22. https://www.montgomeryadvertiser.com.

Macías-Rojas, Patrisia. 2016. *From Deportation to Prison: The Politics of Immigration Enforcement in Post-Civil Rights America*. New York: New York University Press.

Marrow, Helen B., and Tiffany D. Joseph. 2015. "Excluded and Frozen Out: Unauthorised Immigrants' (Non)Access to Care after US Health Care Reform." *Journal of Ethnic and Migration Studies* 41 (14): 2253–73.

Martin, Rachel. 2020. "Why Many Latinos Are Wary of Getting the COVID-19 Vaccine." National Public Radio, December 15. https://www.npr.org.

Martínez-Schuldt, Ricardo D., and Daniel E. Martínez. 2019. "Sanctuary Policies and City-Level Incidents of Violence, 1990 to 2010." *Justice Quarterly* 36 (4): 567–93.

Massoglia, Michael, and William Alex Pridemore. 2015. "Incarceration and Health." *Annual Review of Sociology* 41 (1): 291–310.

McCall, Leslie. 2005. "The Complexity of Intersectionality." *Signs: Journal of Women in Culture and Society* 30 (3): 1771–800.

Meisner, Jason. 2015. "Independent Experts Blast Quality of Medical Care in Illinois Prisons." *Chicago Tribune*, May 19. https://www.chicagotribune.com.

Menjívar, Cecilia. 2011. *Enduring Violence: Ladina Women's Lives in Guatemala*. Berkeley: University of California Press.

Mettler, Suzanne. 2002. "Bringing the State Back in to Civic Engagement: Policy Feedback Effects of the G.I. Bill for World War II Veterans." *American Political Science Review* 96 (2): 351–65.

Mettler, Suzanne, and Joe Soss. 2004. "The Consequences of Public Policy for Democratic Citizenship: Bridging Policy Studies and Mass Politics." *Perspectives on Politics* 2 (1): 55–73.

Metzl, Jonathan M., and Helena Hansen. 2014. "Structural Competency: Theorizing a New Medical Engagement with Stigma and Inequality." *Social Science & Medicine* 103: 126–33.

Michener, Jamila. 2018. *Fragmented Democracy: Medicaid, Federalism, and Unequal Politics*. Cambridge, UK: Cambridge University Press.

Middlemass, Keesha. 2017. *Convicted and Condemned: The Politics and Policies of Prisoner Reentry*. New York: New York University Press.

Milkman, Ruth. 2017. "A New Political Generation: Millennials and the Post-2008 Wave of Protest." *American Sociological Review* 82 (1): 1–31.

Miller, Reuben J. 2021. *Halfway Home: Race, Punishment, and the Afterlife of Mass Incarceration*. Little, Brown.

Miller, Reuben Jonathan. 2014. "Devolving the Carceral State: Race, Prisoner Reentry, and the Micro-Politics of Urban Poverty Management." *Punishment & Society* 16 (3): 305–35.

Mink, Gwendolyn. 1998. *Welfare's End*. Ithaca, NY: Cornell University Press.

Montgomery, James D. 1992. "Job Search and Network Composition: Implications of the Strength-of-Weak-Ties Hypothesis." *American Sociological Review* 57 (5): 586–96.

Nall, Rachel, Kimberly Holland, and Kristeen Cherney. 2018. "The Cost of HIV Treatment." *Healthline*, March 29. https://www.healthline.com.

National Center for Victims of Crime. 2018. "Address Confidentiality Programs." Arlington, VA: National Center for Victims of Crime. http://victimsofcrime.org.

National Women's Law Center. 2017. "Double the Trouble: Health Care Access without the Affordable Care Act or Planned Parenthood." Washington, DC: National Women's Law Center. https://nwlc.org.

Neegaard, Lauran, and Hannah Fingerhut. 2020. "AP-NORC Poll: Only Half in US Want Shots as Vaccine Nears." Associated Press. https://apnews.com.

Nelson, Alondra. 2011. *Body and Soul: The Black Panther Party and the Fight against Medical Discrimination*. Minneapolis: University of Minnesota Press.

Ortega, Alexander N., Hai Fang, Victor H. Perez, John A. Rizzo, Olivia Carter-Pokras, Steven P. Wallace, and Lillian Gelberg. 2007. "Health Care Access, Use of Services, and Experiences among Undocumented Mexicans and Other Latinos." *Archives of Internal Medicine* 167 (21): 2354–60.

Ortega, Alexander N., Hector P. Rodriguez, and Arturo Vargas Bustamante. 2015. "Policy Dilemmas in Latino Health Care and Implementation of the Affordable Care Act." *Annual Review of Public Health* 36: 525–44.

Ortiz, Vikki. 2017. "Shortage of Caregivers for People with Disabilities Intensifies State-wide." *Chicago Tribune*, May 12. https://www.chicagotribune.com.

Pager, Devah. 2003. "The Mark of a Criminal Record." *American Journal of Sociology* 108 (5): 937–75.

Pandey, Erica. 2017. "55 Million People Have Access to Free Birth Control under ACA." *Axios*, October 7. https://www.axios.com.

Parker, Ruth. 2000. "Health Literacy: A Challenge for American Patients and their Health Care Providers." *Health Promotion International* 15 (4): 277–83.

Parreñas, Rhacel. 2015. *Servants of Globalization: Migration and Domestic Work*. Palo Alto, CA: Stanford University Press.

Patel, Kavita, Amy Boutwell, Bradley W. Brockmann, and Josiah D. Rich. 2014. "Integrating Correctional and Community Health Care for Formerly Incarcerated People Who Are Eligible for Medicaid." *Health Affairs* 33 (3): 468–73.

Pear, Robert. 2016. "Health Care Penalty? I'll Take It, Millions Say." *New York Times*, October 26. https://www.nytimes.com.

Pedraza, Franciso I., Vanessa Cruz Nichols, and Alana M. W. LeBrón. 2017. "Cautious Citizenship: The Deterring Effect of Immigration Issue Salience on Health Care Use and Bureaucratic Interactions among Latino US Citizens." *Journal of Health Politics, Policy and Law* 42 (5): 925–60.

Peguero, Anthony A., and Nicole L. Bracy. 2015. "School Order, Justice, and Education: Climate, Discipline Practices, and Dropping Out." *Journal of Research on Adolescence* 25 (3): 412–26.

Pence, Ellen, and Martha McMahon. 1999. "Duluth: A Coordinated Community Response to Domestic Violence." In *The Multi-Agency Approach to Domestic Violence: New Opportunities, Old Challenges?*, edited by Nicola Harwin, Gill Hague, and Ellen Malos, 150–68. London: Whiting & Birch.

Pérez-Escamilla, Rafael, Jonathan Garcia, and David Song. 2010. "Health Care Access among Hispanic Immigrants: ¿Alguien Está Escuchando? [Is Anybody Listening?]." *NAPA Bulletin* 34 (1): 47–67.

Ralph, Laurence. 2015. "Becoming Aggrieved: An Alternative Framework of Care in Black Chicago." *RSF: The Russell Sage Foundation Journal of the Social Sciences* 1 (2): 31–41.

Rape, Abuse & Incest National Network. 2018. "Victims of Sexual Violence Statistics." Washington, DC: Rape, Abuse & Incest National Network. https://www.rainn.org.

Raudenbush, Danielle T. 2020. "Health Care Off the Books: Poverty, Illness, and Strategies for Survival in Urban America." Berkeley: University of California Press.

Rengifo, Andres F., and Morgan Pater. 2017. "Close Call: Race and Gender in Encounters with the Police by Black and Latino/a Youth in New York City." *Sociological Inquiry* 87 (2): 337–61.

Renzetti, Claire M. 1994. "On Dancing with a Bear: Reflections on Some of the Current Debates among Domestic Violence Theorists." *Violence and Victims* 9 (2): 195–200.

Rich, Josiah D., Sarah E. Wakeman, and Samuel L. Dickman. 2011. "Medicine and the Epidemic of Incarceration in the United States." *The New England Journal of Medicine* 364 (22): 2081.

Rios, Victor M. 2011. *Punished: Policing the Lives of Black and Latino Boys*. New York: New York University Press.

———. 2015. "Decolonizing the White Space in Urban Ethnography." *City & Community* 14 (3): 258–61.

———. 2017. *Human Targets: Schools, Police and the Criminalization of Latino Youth*. Chicago: University of Chicago Press.

Risman, B. J. 2009. "From Doing to Undoing: Gender as We Know It." *Gender & Society* 23 (1): 81–84.

Rondini, Ashley C. 2016. "Healing the Hidden Injuries of Class? Redemption Narratives, Aspirational Proxies, and Parents of Low-Income, First-Generation College Students." *Sociological Forum* 31 (1): 96–116.

Rosenthal, Elisabeth. 2013. "The Soaring Cost of a Simple Breath." *New York Times*, October 12. https://www.nytimes.com.

Royner, Julie. 2008. "Health Care's a Big Issue. Who Covers Candidates?" National Public Radio, January 14. https://www.npr.org.

Savage, Terry. 2017. "What to Do if You Can't Afford Obamacare." *Chicago Tribune*. https://www.chicagotribune.com.

Schneider, Anne, and Helen Ingram. 1993. "Social Construction of Target Populations: Implications for Politics and Policy." *American Political Science Review* 87 (2): 334–47.

Scott, Ellen K., Andrew S. London, and Nancy A. Myers. 2002. "Dangerous Dependencies: The Intersection of Welfare Reform and Domestic Violence." *Gender & Society* 16 (6): 878–97.

Seim, Josh. 2017. "The Ambulance: Toward a Labor Theory of Poverty Governance." *American Sociological Review* 82 (3): 451–75.

Sered, Susan Starr. 2005. *Uninsured in America Life and Death in the Land of Opportunity*. Berkeley: University of California Press.

Shim, Janet K. 2010. "Cultural Health Capital: A Theoretical Approach to Understanding Health Care Interactions and the Dynamics of Unequal Treatment." *Journal of Health and Social Behavior* 51 (1): 1–15.

Siddiqi, Arjumand A., Susan Wang, Kelly Quinn, Quynh C. Nguyen, and Antony Dennis Christy. 2016. "Racial Disparities in Access to Care under Conditions of Universal Coverage." *American Journal of Preventive Medicine* 50 (2): 220–25.

Small, Mario Luis. 2009. *Unanticipated Gains: Origins of Network Inequality in Everyday Life*. Oxford, UK: Oxford University Press.

Smith, Robert. 2006. *Mexican New York: Transnational Lives of New Immigrants*. Berkeley: University of California Press.

Sonier, J., M. H. Boudreaux, and L. A. Blewett. 2013. "Medicaid 'Welcome-Mat' Effect of Affordable Care Act Implementation Could Be Substantial." *Health Affairs* 32 (7): 1319–25.

Soss, Joe. 2000. *Unwanted Claims: The Politics of Participation in the U.S. Welfare System*. Ann Arbor: University of Michigan Press.

Soss, Joe. 2002. *Unwanted Claims: The Politics of Participation in the U.S. Welfare System*. Paperback ed. Ann Arbor: University of Michigan Press.

Soss, Joe, Richard C. Fording, and Sanford F. Schram. 2011. *Disciplining the Poor: Neoliberal Paternalism and the Persistent Power of Race*. Chicago: University of Chicago Press.

Soss, Joe, and Vesla Weaver. 2017. "Police Are Our Government: Politics, Political Science, and the Policing of Race–Class Subjugated Communities." *Annual Review of Political Science* 20: 565–91.

Starr, Paul. 2017. *The Social Transformation of American Medicine: The Rise of a Sovereign Profession and the Making of a Vast Industry*. Basic Books.

State of Illinois. 2018. "Candidate's Guide." Edited by State Board of Elections. https://elections.il.gov.

Stuart, Forrest. 2016. *Down, Out, and Under Arrest: Policing and Everyday Life in Skid Row*. Chicago: University of Chicago Press.

Tabachnick, Cara. 2014. "Obamacare for Ex-Inmates: Is Health Insurance an Antidote to Crime?" *The Christian Science Monitor*, July 27. https://www.csmonitor.com.

Taubman, Sarah L., Heidi L. Allen, Bill J. Wright, Katherine Baicker, and Amy N. Finkelstein. 2014. "Medicaid Increases Emergency-Department Use: Evidence from Oregon's Health Insurance Experiment." *Science* 343 (6168): 263–68.

Telles, Edward E., and Vilma Ortiz. 2008. *Generations of Exclusion: Mexican-Americans, Assimilation, and Race*. New York: Russell Sage Foundation.

Trouille, David, and Iddo Tavory. 2019. "Shadowing: Warrants for Intersituational Variation in Ethnography." *Sociological Methods & Research* 48 (3): 534–60.

US Bureau of Labor Statistics. 2019. "Union Workers More Likely than Nonunion Workers to Have Healthcare Benefits in 2019." *TED: The Economics Daily*, October 28. https://www.bls.gov.

US Census Bureau. 2020. "2016–2019 American Community Survey 3-year Public Use Microdata Samples."

Vargas, Edward D. 2015. "Immigration Enforcement and Mixed-Status Families: The Effects of Risk of Deportation on Medicaid Use." *Children and Youth Services Review* 57: 83–89.

Vargas, Nicholas. 2018. "Racial Expropriation in Higher Education: Are Whiter Hispanic Serving Institutions More Likely to Receive Minority Serv-

ing Institution Funds?" *Socius* 4: 1–12. https://journals.sagepub.com/doi.
pdf/10.1177/2378023118794077

Vargas, Robert. 2019. "Gangstering Grants: Bringing Power to Collective Efficacy Theory." *City & Community* 18 (1): 369–91.

Vargas Bustamante, Arturo, Hai Fang, John A. Rizzo, and Alexander N. Ortega. 2009. "Understanding Observed and Unobserved Health Care Access and Utilization Disparities Among U.S. Latino Adults." *Medical Care Research and Review* 66 (5): 561–77.

Vasquez, Jessica M. 2011. *Mexican Americans across Generations: Immigrant Families, Racial Realities*. New York: New York University Press.

Vega, William A., Michael A. Rodriguez, and Elisabeth Gruskin. 2009. "Health Disparities in the Latino Population." *Epidemiologic Reviews* 31 (1): 99–112.

Villa-Torres, Laura, Paul J. Fleming, and Clare Barrington. 2015. "Engaging Men as Promotores de Salud: Perceptions of Community Health Workers among Latino Men in North Carolina." *Journal of Community Health* 40 (1): 167–74.

Villalón, Roberta. 2010. *Violence against Latina Immigrants: Citizenship, Inequality, and Community*. New York: New York University Press.

Viruell-Fuentes, Edna A., Patricia Y. Miranda, and Sawsan Abdulrahim. 2012. "More than Culture: Structural Racism, Intersectionality Theory, and Immigrant Health." *Social Science & Medicine* 75 (12): 2099–106.

Walker, Michael L. 2016. "Race Making in a Penal Institution." *American Journal of Sociology* 121 (4): 1051–78.

Wallace, Steven P., and Valentine M. Villa. 2003. "Equitable Health Systems: Cultural and Structural Issues for Latino Elders." *American Journal of Law & Medicine* 29 (2–3): 247.

Walsh, Dylan. 2017. "Does Bad Health Care Constitute Cruel and Unusual Punishment?" *The Atlantic*, June 17. https://www.theatlantic.com.

Walter, Nicolas, Philippe Bourgois, and H. Margarita Loinaz. 2004. "Masculinity and Undocumented Labor Migration: Injured Latino Day laborers in San Franciso." *Social Science and Medicine* 59 (6): 1159–68.

Walter, Shoshana. 2010. "Officers See More Sick and Elderly Selling Prescription Drugs." *New York Times*, September 18. https://www.nytimes.com.

Washington, Harriet A. 2006. *Medical Apartheid: The Dark History of Medical Experimentation on Black Americans from Colonial Times to the Present*. New York: Doubleday.

Watkins-Hayes, Celeste. 2009. *The New Welfare Bureaucrats: Entanglements of Race, Class, and Policy Reform*. Chicago: University of Chicago Press.

Western, Bruce. 2006. *Punishment and Inequality in America*. New York: Russell Sage Foundation.

———. 2018. *Homeward: Life in the Year After Prison*. New York: Russell Sage Foundation.

Wilper, Andrew P., Steffie Woolhandler, J. Wesley Boyd, Karen E. Lasser, Danny McCormick, David H. Bor, and David U. Himmelstein. 2009. "The Health and Health

Care of US Prisoners: Results of a Nationwide Survey." *American Journal of Public Health* 99 (4): 666–72.

Wogan, J. B. 2016. "Who's an Employee? The Uber Important Question of Today's Economy." *Governing*, May 24. http://www.governing.com.

Zambrana, Ruth E., and Bonnie Thornton Dill. 2006. "Disparities in Latina Health: An Intersectional Analysis." In *Gender, Race, Class, and Health: Intersectional Approaches*, edited by Amy J. Schulz and L. Mullings, 192–227. San Francisco, CA: Jossey-Bass.

Zamudio, Maria I. 2020. "How Promotoras Are Fighting Vaccine Conspiracies in Chicago's Latino Communities." *WBEZ*. http://www.wbez.org.

Zarate, Maria Estela, and Ronald Gallimore. 2005. "Gender Differences in Factors Leading to College Enrollment: A Longitudinal Analysis of Latina and Latino Students." *Harvard Educational Review* 75 (4): 383–408.

Zelman, Walter A. 2014. "College Campuses Are Fertile Ground for Promoting Obamacare." *Los Angeles Times*, July 27. https://www.latimes.com.

Zuberi, Tukufu. 2001. *Thicker Than Blood: How Racial Statistics Lie*. Minneapolis: University of Minnesota Press.

INDEX

Page numbers in *italics* indicate Figures and Tables

ABOUT THE AUTHOR

ROBERT VARGAS is Associate Professor of Sociology at the University of Chicago. He is the author of the multi-award-winning *Wounded City: Violent Turf Wars in a Chicago Barrio* and a recipient of the Career Award from the National Science Foundation.